YOUR COMPLETE MOTIVATIONAL GUIDE TO

MOTIVATIONAL
WEIGHT LOSS

- **GILBERT** QUINONES

For more information on content such as this visit
MotivationalLove.com. This book is intended to help
turn the hope, dreams, and desires of all the special
people in this world so that they can be free from the
limitations of their weight.

The information provided in this book is for informational purposes only and is not intended as a substitute for advice from your physician or other health care professional or any information contained on or in any product label or packaging. The information and claims made in this book have not been evaluated by the United States Food and Drug Administration and are not approved to diagnose, treat, cure, or prevent disease. Check with your doctor before changing your diet. The author is not a trained medical professional. All references to manufacture product information, labels, and web addresses are provided for informational purposes only and cannot be relied upon for accuracy as product information, labels, and web addresses change from time to time.

For information about custom editions, special sales, premium and corporate purchases please contact sales@motivationallove.com

For more information visit :**www.MotivationalLove.com**

Your Complete Motivation Guide to Weight Loss

This book is dedicated to all those who struggle with their weight and want to live life to the fullest.

MOTIVATIONAL WEIGHT LOSS
Gilbert Quinones
"Your Complete Motivational Weight Loss Guide"

Contents

Contents *(Continued)*:

—

An Important Note from Gilbert Quinones:

Having spent over 10 years of my life being obese, I can tell you that it does something to someone. Waking up not having the energy to live life or do nothing but think of eating puts you stuck in a rut. This stuck in the rut phase can take away from what life has to offer you. Although success comes in all shapes and forms it is the satisfaction of the transformation process that affects one's mental health to achieve new things in life. These are the times that all the money and power do not mean anything since it makes you realize what is the point if you can not enjoy it.

Life has given me everything I could possibly need and now it is time I can give back to you.
The techniques and principles you are about to read here will take you on a mind transformation journey. This book is your first-class ticket to clear your mind of all thoughts of negativity and begin your path to your personal fitness destination.

If you felt this book had an impact on your life then recommend it to others as well. It will make a difference in the lives of the people you care about and how you can help them.

" 10% of all proceeds from this book are donated to the Special Olympics to help touch the lives of special children & adults in our world. Thank you for choosing to give back."

-Gilbert Quinones

Preface

What You Should Know

Short, sweet, and effective, if you are looking for weight loss motivation then this book is all you need. What this book does is takes the many intricacies in the medical field of fitness and simplifies them so everyday people understand how the mind works when trying to lose weight. By reading these chapters your mind will begin a transformation. You will begin a psychological journey of thoughts that will give you the mental strength to turn your mind into a weight-loss machine.

This book is the perfect size of content to absorb effectively, keep you engaged and not overwhelm you.

Reference back to it from time to time to gain the mental visuals and motivation you need. If you ever fall off the track just review the chapters needed to gain the ability to see clearly and maintain your focus.

Let the content absorb you and you will achieve the body you've always desired. You will never think or feel the same way again when it comes to losing weight. You will now feel abundant with motivation and empowered.

Start your fitness goals and start losing weight beginning right now this very moment you read these words. Every single one of these chapters will play a key role to give you the motivational knowledge you need on your weight loss journey.

Hang on to your seats because it's time to change your life forever.

Introductory

The Mind Controls the Body

The Lemon

Try this mental experiment. Imagine the freshest juiciest yellow lemon you have ever seen. Visualize it. Imagine taking a knife and cutting it in half to the point it is so fresh lemon juice squirts out and runs down your palm. You can smell the fresh lemon scent just as you open it in two pieces. Imagine taking one of the halves up to your mouth and bite into it sucking as hard as you can as you quench the thirst of soaking pure lemon juice straight to your mouth. It will make your mouth pucker and your face will have the sourest face you can imagine. At the very thought of this process of reading these words, you might notice your saliva glands right now are drenching with natural juices just by the thought of biting into a fresh lemon. This is a sample of how effective the mind can control the body and it works in all aspects of our lives especially with the weight loss process. The problem is that most people tend to jump into what they are told to do and forget about the source that controls the body's actions. Learn to train your mind to think like a weight-loss machine and you will become the most effective dieter around resulting in the body you desire.

Every chapter in this book is a key element to your fitness goals.

...introduction continued.

The mind controls the body so feed the mind first. There are plenty of books that tell you what to eat along with tips on how to lose weight. Have you ever taken the time to read the many intricate details of an average weight loss or diet book? You will find that most of them are simply all logic, eat this and do that. For example, you may have experienced reading weight loss material in detail. You then follow the structure of the diet and eating healthy food choices that resulted in you losing weight however, you may have gained the weight back. How do you prevent this from happening again? What is the initial phase that forces us to take action to follow better-eating habits? What determines if the logical decisions of good food choices are practiced on a daily basis? Why does this seem to be such a hard process? Why can't we just simply go to the fridge and grab the nonfat, no sugar plain yogurt rather than grabbing the delicious ice cream without thinking twice?

For some, this is just not that easy. Before these dieting decisions can be carried out it starts with our thoughts first. It starts with our motivation to lose weight and our abilities to get motivated. That is what this book is about! It is to help train your brain to make the right choices when you face these decisions on a daily basis. It starts in the mind.

Feed The Mind 1st

Ultimately the body will reciprocate with the mind however, you have to start by feeding your mind first before you start to feed your stomach to reach your fitness goals.

This is why so many have such a difficult time reaching their fitness goals. It is like trying to skip over the most important process. Most people know where they want to go. They know the type of body they would like to achieve and have clear intentions of what they desire. However, just because you have a destination does not mean you have a map to get there. Have you ever stopped to ask for directions to a location? In the olden days before GPS and smartphones, many people were always asking for directions. When you would stop at a convenience store to ask for directions the person tells you to go here, turn left at the 3rd block, take another right, and go about 3 miles and so on and it will be on the left side. You then get in the car confused trying to remember everything you were just told. This is sometimes the reality of the fitness world. Experts are telling you everything to do and what not to do leaving you confused and lost.

It all comes out too fast and they came across as knowledgeable because most likely they have been to that destination before. This is the reason personal trainers are generally very fit and knowledgeable. They have already been to their destination and know how to get there.

What if you could know where you are going as if you have already been there? What if you were already at your fitness goals? What if you could go back in time, and tell a younger version of yourself exactly how to give your own self the directions you can understand? You can by feeding your mind first and reading this book.

This book will be your GPS map to your fitness destination.

Chapter 1

First - Which Motivation Level Are You?

Level Up!

This chapter simplifies the different motivation levels of people when it comes to fitness. It also shows how they may maneuver in the different paths of their lives when it comes to the decisions they make for their fitness based on these motivation levels. It also creates much controversy however in retrospect is never discussed due to the sensitivity of some of the topics. Understanding the reasons and different motivational levels will be to your benefit. It will help you so that you can place where you are currently and where you want to be. Understand each level of motivation before making the decision of your final destination of fitness.

Comfort Levels

MOTIVATIONAL LEVEL UP CHART!

Motivation Level 3	Motivation Level 2	Motivation Level 1
		Thinks About Fitness often
	Thinks about Fitness on and off . But strives To Be Fit	Has Exercise Ritual
Does not Generally Think about Fitness		
Rarely Exercises	Exercises occasionally But still strives	Has a Dieting Plan for A Lifestyle
Usually Eats Whatever Think About	On and Off Dieting	

Motivation Level 1 - Extremely Motivated

This person is extremely motivated and fitness is a high priority to them. The majority of the time is generally a single person. Fitness is a ritual in their life.

Motivation Level 2 - Normal Motivation

This person is fairly motivated about health and fitness and occasionally drifts back and forth. Usually wants to be fit but does not want it bad enough. Fitness creates friction in their life.

Motivation Level 3 - Not Motivated

This person is not motivated. This is a growing population and is becoming more accepted in society as time progresses. Fitness is not thought of in their life.

Determine which level of motivation you are at. After you have decided which motivation level you are read forward about each of the different levels. Understand how each of these people has their priorities in their life and why. Then make the decision of which level you want to be on after you understand clearly what each one's priorities are. Once you understand them you can make a more decisive decision that will be embedded in your mind of what level you want to be on and stay at.

Understanding Motivational Levels

Motivation Level 3 - Not Motivated

This is not a bad person. Eating right or exercising is just simply not a priority to them. For whatever reason, they may have not been taught nor did they have a healthy lifestyle role model in their life. Does this make it right? For example, if your role model did not teach you how to treat others with respect would it be okay for you to grow up and treat people the same way your role model taught you? Absolutely not. That is the reason we have to make the decisions as good human beings to make the right choices as we grow and develop the awareness of being healthy.

If you were never taught how to have self-respect for yourself the way you do for others then now is the time for you to start respecting your body. Adapting to a healthy lifestyle is essential for many reasons.

- Self Respect
- Keeping healthy for our loved ones
- Being able to provide physical protection for our loved ones if needed, man or woman
- Live a much more fulfilling life and longevity

The majority of the people in the Level 3 Motivation category are generally in a secure relationship or marriage. They generally encounter in sexual relations through their secure relationship. If a level 3 motivated person is single then it's possible they may have low self-esteem or have given up on finding a partner. If they are not sexually active then they may have accepted the fact to not have sex as often.

Motivation Level 2 - Normal Motivation

This person will diet occasionally and will put effort into exercising in trends. They will seasonally be seen at the gym and they realize a healthy lifestyle needs to be more of a priority in their life. The majority of these people in this range of motivation are married or are in a secure relationship. They eat right periodically. They are occasionally sexually active or are very sexual active generally through secure relationships or marriage. However, there are some people with this level of motivation who are not as sexually active focus on fitness will usually be those times of sexual inactivity.

Motivation Level 1 - Extremely Motivated

This person has adapted to eating well and exercising as a lifestyle. It is not necessarily a chore for them since it is what they know. Their motivation factor is fairly high since being healthy is a priority for them. They are generally single. That does not mean someone can be motivated at this level and not be married. Anybody can be extremely motivated. It just means that statistically speaking the majority of these people are single. Since the majority of the Motivation Level 1 people are not involved in secure relationships, for them to be sexually active they normally engage in social activities with others for potential partners to engage in sexual activities consistently. This is part of an instinct that is always working in the back of the subconscious mind of these individuals usually without them knowing. Since these people are generally also fit, their desire for sexual intercourse is greater than the average person for the following reasons:

1) Confidence: They feel better about themselves and have the confidence to be proactive in social environments.

2) Opportunities: They have more opportunities coming at them since they are generally more attractive due to their fitness lifestyle.

3) Health: Their bodies reciprocate with their minds and they feel better internally resulting in their body's to have the ability to perform at optimum levels for sexual activity. When the organs and the body's systems are at prime levels one's abilities to include the bodies natural hormones will be at a peak level to perform. Simply put, being in a healthy state can affect a person's total sexual desires and performances to take better care of themselves subconsciously.

Affecting Your Health
Affecting Your Social Life
Affecting Your Abilities

Understand the Disadvantages/Advantages

Take the time to understand the repercussions of not being healthy. Understand what in your life is being affected by not having the body you want. By taking the time to understand them you are assisting your mind to set up the foundation to renovate your new motivational level. Once you understand exactly what the disadvantages are you will be able to focus on the positive outcomes of making the changes. Almost everything we do in life is either a step to avoid pain or a step to move closer to pleasure. When you have an understanding of the disadvantages and advantages you can make decisions based on the purest simplified form of thought to move in the direction of avoiding the pain and move towards the pleasures in life.

You can do it.

Crystal Clear Vision

Do you have a clear vision of the body you want? Do you want to be high school skinny, slim, athletic? Thoughts become things. Everything we do starts with a thought. It starts with a vision. Once you have a clear vision you have an objective. You now understand where you are and where you want to go. How you get there will soon begin to unfold but it will all start with a simple thought. It is this thought of your crystal clear vision of what you are going to achieve that will put your mind into action. It is this visualization that will carry out your actions to what you desire. Don't overly obsess over it daily. Realize it is going to take some time and find a balance to gradually make changes and transform your physique as your body is meant to look. Start with the mind power and start envisioning the body you want.

Vision Your Worth

Most people have a standard of acceptance of what they consider beautiful is on the outside. Our inner beauty can be seen by getting to know us and is many times overlooked because our physical beauty sometimes shields us from the outside world preventing people from getting to know us on the inside. The standard of what people consider to be physically beautiful in the world is all cliche and changes over time.

Marilyn Monroe is an example of how society viewed beauty back in the 1940s-1950s. Looking into the glamorous eyes of a Marilyn Monroe portrait you can feel the old souls during that time and see the beauty they saw through their eyes. But as time has passed this is no longer the commonly accepted standard of physical beauty. Even the weight standard of models has changed over the years and what was once the perceived standard of beauty evolves and changes. Modern-day models that look nothing like the past prove that. This illustrates how as a society we have a standard of physiological beauty that changes.

Most people in the present time have a standard of what they consider to be physically beautiful. You also most likely deep down have a perception of the physical beauty of what is acceptable for your own body whether if you are happy with how you look or desire to look better. Whether you are already in shape or not, you deserve to feel as beautiful as you want. If you feel beautiful on the inside then vision your worth. Visualize your inner beauty so that it begins to reflect on your outer beauty. When you realize your worth on the inside, it makes it easier to feel the reasons on why you need to take care of yourself. Visualize your worth on the inside, so you can release your outer fitness beauty on the outside.

Decide If You Will Make The Climb

Understand this one thing when deciding to make the change to transforming your body

"If it was easy, everyone would be doing it. Do I have what it takes to do what may not be easy and do I want the reward bad enough?"

The one thing that separates successful people is the decisions they make to sacrifice. With this sacrifice, there is great reward. The select few who create the vision, crave the reward, and sacrifice, are the ones who achieve. No one said losing weight was necessarily going to be an easy process, however, when you can get a clear image of the percentage of people that have succeeded you gain perspective. You will see that these people simply made decisions to sacrifice. It's similar to the many physical achievements in life that different athletes make. The first person to climb Mount Everest had an extraordinary act of human abilities that was unheard of. Once one person achieved this then many came to follow. Now the human minds of others do not doubt if it is possible. They know it is possible and they set a path of the clear vision in their minds when going through the struggle.

Know what is possible. Realize what makes people different if they succeed. Understand the simple fact that if it were easy everyone would do it. Mentally climb your own Mount Everest. Once you get there along with your desired body, the feeling of confidence and the feeling of self-accomplishment will make you feel like you are on top of the world.

It is the greatest feeling ever.

ACTION STEPS:

1) Understand Your Motivation Level- Figure out where you are at in your motivation level. Once you have a clear understanding of the different levels of motivation of people and what drives them you can better place yourself to gain perspective. When we understand the reasons of "what" and "why", we can better assess ourselves to put a valuation of our own motivation level and determine how we can go to the next level of motivation. Level Up!

2) Create Your Crystal Clear Vision

3) Decide to Make The Climb

CONCLUSION

Weight loss is a state of mind of controlling yourself and your surroundings.

OVERHEATING AT SEAWORLD - Trying to enjoy the little things.

It was the peak of the Texas summer in 2004 and I was taking my family to SeaWorld. I was nearly 300lbs. The heat was unbearable at 104 degrees and it was not comfortable to stand outside in those temperatures for an average person let alone for an obese person.

We were just getting done watching our second show(the dolphins). I remember seeing people having spray bottles with little fans on them and I couldn't wait to get my hands on one! As the show was over we fought the crowd and waited in the heat to get out of the dolphin stadium. It was an unbearable torture and all I wanted to do was find an air-conditioned place to sit down. It was time to go to the next show when I soon realized that I was not capable of continuing to walk.

This was an extremely crucial moment in my life that I did not want to admit out loud. I could not finish the shows we planned to see at SeaWorld because I was out of breath and out of shape. My 6-year-old son Julius gazed up into my sweaty face and asked me sincerely. "Dad, are you going to be able to make the next show?" As much as I wanted to tell him yes I could not walk in the heat anymore. He was so excited and was ready for more entertainment but it was hard for me to keep up. It was a time of reflection for myself and what I had let myself become.

This eye-opening experience was the catalyst and basis for my motivation. If I couldn't enjoy the little things with my family then what is the point? It was in that moment I knew I had to change...

I made a dramatic physical change using the principles discussed in this book.

Find what motivates you, so you can enjoy the little things.

Chapter 2

The Hunger Pain Drug

Cravings vs Good Food Choices

The addiction of food. Hunger is the drug.

How to control the cravings.

You have to learn to battle the addiction by not letting the drug craving overcome you.

How do you do this? It may seem so hard to make the right choices when so many foods taste so good.

The key to battling the cravings is quite simple.

Try to battle the cravings before it is too late!

Meaning, battle the cravings before the cravings get too strong. Don't try to make the best food decisions on an empty stomach.

Unbearable Cravings - Our Natural Instincts
The following illustration is a perfect example of how hunger affects our ability to make the right decisions in the animal kingdom.

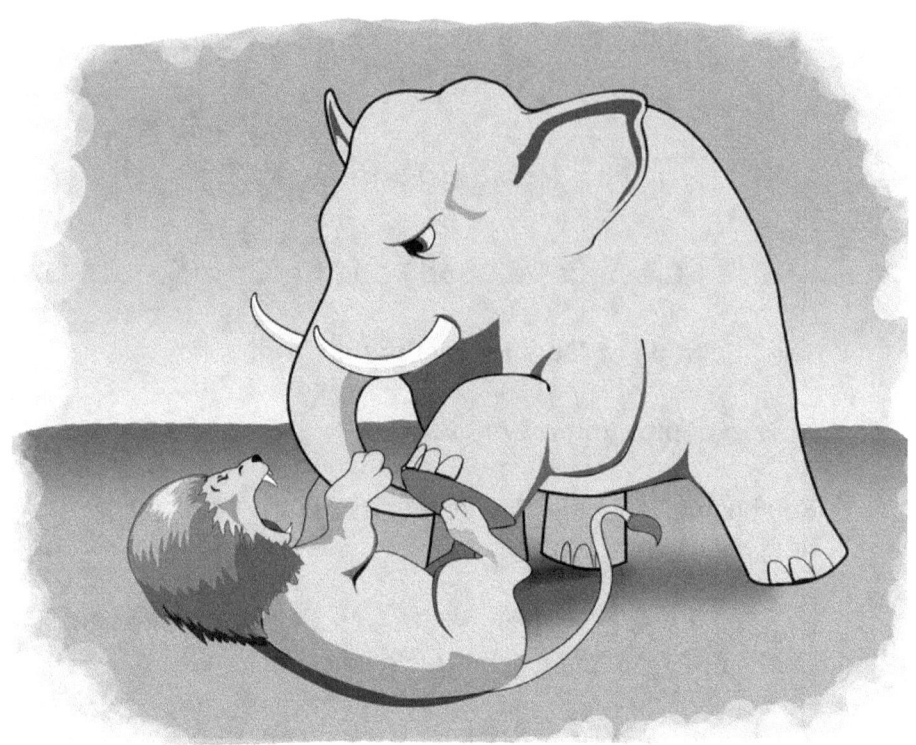

Lions weigh approximately 400-500 pounds. However, elephants can grow over 8 tons. This means that as a full-size adult elephant the animal is so enormous that one leg can easily weigh over one thousand pounds. The elephant is so massive it can easily crush the predator lion if the lion makes one single mistake. However, when droughts come in Africa and food is scarce, lions become desperate and hunger kicks in. This results in them making very rare illogical decisions based on this hunger and once in awhile lions will perform an act against nature by attacking a full-grown adult elephant. Most of the time they do not succeed and risk their fate of being crushed from the elephant as a result of their unbearable hunger.

We as humans many times every day take this risk in life as our natural instinct of hunger kicks in. Every time we let hunger get out of control we risk slowly coming closer to killing ourselves with everyday bad food choices. Have you ever woke up in the morning and left in a hurry by not eating breakfast? You go the entire day and barely get a chance to grab a late lunch. Then lunch passes and when you finally get a chance to grab something you are starving. What is the first thing you think about? Do you want to run to the closest Subway and eat a light 6 inch veggie sandwich on wheat bread with no cheese or do want to go to the nearest drive-thru and grab the burger combo with fries and a drink? If you are extremely hungry and have missed breakfast and lunch most likely you will give in to the hamburger.

This is called unbearable cravings and if you let it happen it will continue to crash your diet day after day killing you slowly. Do not take the risk if food is not scarce.

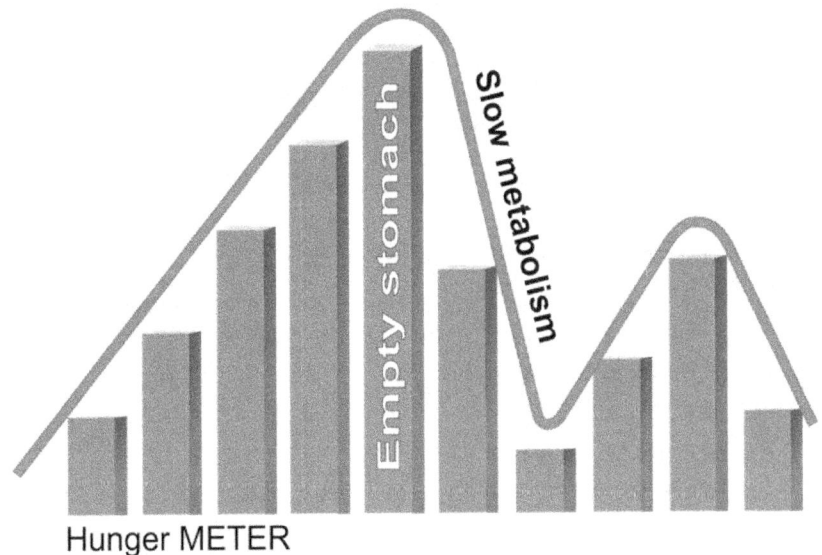

Hunger METER

Naturally, it is easier to control the foods you eat when you are not on a totally empty stomach. When you stay fed with good food choices, this is when you become accustomed to eating better. Soon this turns into a habit and then the habit turns into progress. It is such a good feeling because you feel your body becoming healthier as well.

When you are not starving it is easier to eat foods that do not taste as good since your natural cravings are not as high for sugars and natural energy. For example, when you are hungry your blood sugar is low so your body naturally craves sugars and simple carbs as fuel. It is normal to naturally desire this energy boost with these foods. Think about how hard is it for you to battle your cravings for junk food during this time.

Understand your natural cravings and how they work so that you can take the measures needed to make adjustments in your eating routine to stay fed. Make sure you DO NOT go on an empty stomach ever. Battle cravings of junk food by avoiding hunger pains.

THE ENVIRONMENT OF CRAVINGS

Natural Cravings from your surroundings.

There is a mimic concept referred to as mirror neurons. This is a hard craving to deal with but if you are prepared you will overcome it. A mirror neuron is the act of the animal instinct for us to copy the actions of another person's actions subconsciously. This can be a facial expression, scratching an itch on your nose, or any type of animal act when we observe it from another.

You may recall moments throughout your life to where you are minding your own business then someone appears with a bag of fresh food that smells very delicious. Now all of a sudden you are hungry. This is called the mirror neuron effect that's going on subconsciously without us realizing it. You are not necessarily hungry and if you were only slightly hungry your hunger is now magnified because of the image and the smell of food is magnifying your cravings. This is one of the most difficult things to control since you do not have control over your peer's food choices, however, remember you can control your environment. It will be something you have to talk about to your peers that are in your environment to help support you. Ask for their assistance to help you reach your fitness goals and try to prevent yourself from being in these environments that cause cravings. It sounds so simplistic, but the brain will eventually stop craving what it does not think about.

Use Mirror Neurons to Your Advantage

These mirror neurons that magnify your cravings of hunger can also be used to magnify your motivation for fitness. For example, mirror neurons for the desire to be in excellent shape can be magnified when going to fitness facilities and seeing others in extreme shape. It is natural to desire to be as attractive as others in your environment therefore this can be to your advantage if you control your environment to magnify your cravings for the body you seek. Environments affect us like a contagious virus. Stay in the environments that you want to be affected by and catch the fitness disease. It's the best, healthiest virus you can get.

The fact that mirror neurons can subconsciously be

controlled this is to your advantage if you put yourself in the environments you want to become part of the subconscious mind will begin to take over without you even realizing it.

ACTION STEPS:

1) Battle Cravings by Avoiding Hunger Pains - When you are having unbearable hunger pains it's generally by choice of routine. Give yourself the upper hand and keep your stomach slightly full with healthy food choices and eventually you will learn to beat the food craving drug.

2) Consistently Keep Good Foods in Your Body - Remember you are keeping your body's natural energy high to prevent the natural cravings of junk food.

3) Take control of your surroundings and realize the decision is yours - Understand how the craving process works when in front of people so you do not give into it. Good friends will help you with your goals.

CONCLUSION

When you reach your weight loss goals you will achieve a feeling of success. What makes successful people stand out from the rest of everyone else is that they have a clear realization that they decide to be successful. When you realize that the only person that makes this decision is you, you will make all the decisions you need to reach your goals. This applies to business, careers, or prospering your family to live a happy life. It is us who controls our environment, what we eat, what we do, and what we will do.

Realize that you are the one and start controlling your

decisions now and beat the hunger pain drug.

A TICKING TIME BOMB - Life or death?

It was the summer of 2006. I was sitting in my office at my desk and was going through different websites on Google to see where our competitors were ranking. The internet had hit big and played a major factor in a company's success. I remember always being afraid I wouldn't make enough money for my family and that my home would be foreclosed on, even sometimes having nightmares about it. This fear motivated me to always be working.

I was so caught up in my work that I had forgotten that I applied for life insurance a couple of months before. I had just purchased our second franchise and was staying busy running both operations. The business was doing well and I wanted to leave my family in security in case something happened to me. I remember one of my business associates Michael McGehee saying, "Gilbert you don't want to be like Sam Walton... make all this money and die early." Although life insurance was not a complete solution it seemed like it would be an extra security blanket.

Since I applied for a higher insurance benefit the company needed to do a basic test to ensure that I was not a high risk. They came out to my office a few weeks earlier to take a blood sample, weight, and measurements. I did not think anything of it. Although I was overweight, I figured that I had youth on my side. I figured I was only 27 and they would not deny me since I was young. I was wrong. I remember being at my desk as one of my employees delivered me my mail and I saw it was a letter from the insurance company. Expecting to open a letter of approval it was a check. The check was for a refund along with a letter notifying me of my blood test. The test confirmed that I had high cholesterol, blood pressure, classified as obese, and was considered a very high risk. I was denied life insurance. I was only 27.

I was too involved in work and making money and neglected my health. I was a ticking time bomb that was at risk of having a heart attack and losing everything that I worked for. This was the real foreclosure notice. It was a new realization of foreclosure on life and I needed to do some catching up on my health or else my body was about to be repossessed. I then realized that everything I worked for meant nothing if I was dead. It was at that moment, I had to decide what was important to me.

From this point on I recorded all the principles I have used over the years to get in shape. Many people would not have had the ability or resources to take the time to write a book, however, I was fortunate enough to be able to lock myself in a room for several months. Dieting, exercising, and then finding the best way to put these principles into words on the mental approach I took is all listed here.

I consider obesity a mental disease that anyone can suffer from but nearly anyone can cure themselves.

Whether it's realizing that you are a ticking time bomb or just simply wanting to lose a few extra pounds to feel good about yourself. I hope you gain clarity with whatever you have going on in your life to realize that sometimes neglecting your health can mean life or death in the long run.

Take time to reflect on yourself, practice self-health and in your busy world choose "life".

Chapter 3

Two Steps Forward, Never Two Steps Back

Do you remember when you were a kid in the backseat of a vehicle asking, "are we there yet?", "are we there yet?" Isn't it funny when we're kids how we just want to know the progress of our destination? When we are children we don't have clarity of the progress we are making and all we can do is keep asking. We're too young to read a map or GPS. We just sit in the back seat and wait. Not being aware of progress leads to uncertainty, which then leads to discouragement. When we start new eating habits we need to have awareness of the progress we are making. By utilizing a weekly step system, it can give you the clear focus you need for your progress.

Have you ever swam a long-distance? Swimming is an example of not having awareness of the distance you are covering. Sometimes you need to poke your head out of the water to see the great distance you covered. The reason for this is because it takes a tremendous amount of effort for us to be submerged in the water and our bodies to swim. This is the same for starting a new fitness regiment. It takes a lot of effort and you sometimes need to have your head poked out of the water to see how much distance you are covering. The weekly step system is recommended to follow so that you have some kind of perspective on the distance you are covering.

The same way a map or GPS gives you perspective for your estimated time of arrival the weekly step system will work similarly. Everything is about the numbers. Sports statistics, production levels at work, and anything else we achieve always has a measurement of progress. By many people not having any kind of map to achieve their goal is bound to get lost. This is the reason for many that fail at dieting. Know where you are at and where you are going. Use the weekly step system for measurements of your fitness progress.

What Is A STEP

Envision a step as a day of progress that you made to eat right and exercise. It is the day you decided you were going to go into a calorie deficit and not allow your fitness goals to get off track. If you are not familiar with the term calorie deficit, it is simply a day that your body burns more calories than it consumes. This can be done either by eating less, exercise or a combination of both. Therefore a step would be a day you accomplished this objective.

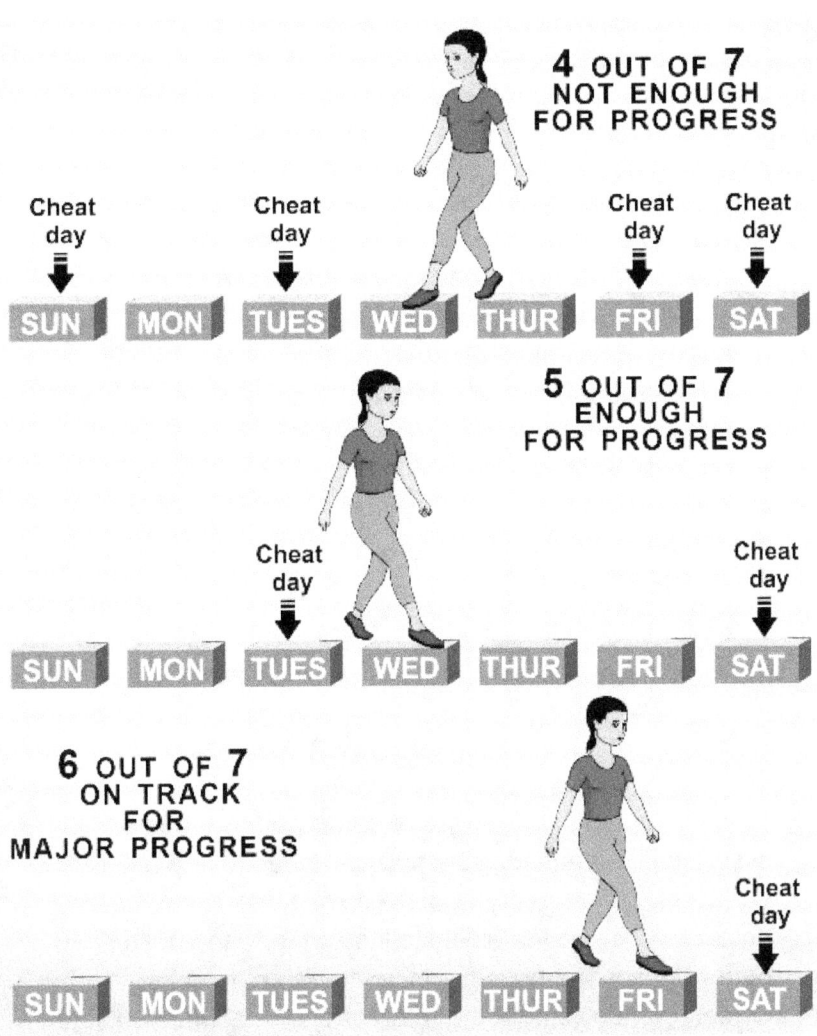

4 OUT OF **7**
NOT ENOUGH
FOR PROGRESS

Cheat day — SUN
Cheat day — MON
Cheat day — FRI
Cheat day — SAT

5 OUT OF **7**
ENOUGH
FOR PROGRESS

Cheat day — TUES
Cheat day — SAT

6 OUT OF **7**
ON TRACK
FOR
MAJOR PROGRESS

Cheat day — SAT

Your 7-day week process is your 7-day point step process. You should be making at least six steps out of the 7 steps per week during your weekly regimen. Imagine the first day of the week on Sunday is step one to your 7-step process. If you diet and exercise correctly throughout the week perfectly and crash on Friday you will probably be okay. You will have just taken only one step backward. However, if you crashed Thursday, Friday, and Saturday then technically you have walked forward four steps and took three steps back. Therefore, what may appear as an entire week of progress was only one step of progress.

People that are on Motivational Level 1 will generally take at least six steps every single week. They realize that it is pointless to take two steps forward then two steps back.

If time only progressed forward by the days we ate right then most people would not make it to Saturday. Every week try to get through your steps without taking more than one step back.

If you are walking and you took two steps backward for every two steps forward you will never get where you need to go. Think of this concept daily and visualize the step technique on as you are going through your week.

Practice Your Fitness Step System Weekly

Practice by definition is the repeated performance or systematic exercise for the purpose of acquiring a skill or proficiency. With every great skill we achieve, requires practice. Gaining the ability to lose weight and build a better body is not necessarily something the average person can do without the effort of practice. Many talented people in today's world gained their traits from the systematic discipline of practice. Envision a professional basketball player. They gain their skills over a period of time and become effective in their profession. Without going through this discipline of practice they will not achieve their goals. Think of your step technique as your practice. Every day you gain the ability to get closer to achieving the body you desire. You might take one day a week off of practice, however, maintain your skills as a result of your weekly practice.

Start taking your steps and practice daily.

Play To Win

Write down what you eat as an additional measurement of progress. When we exercise we measure how much distance we cover, how many reps we did or how many sets we completed. Everything is about the numbers. In sports, it's about the statistics. In business, it's about the profit and loss statements and for investors to make strategic decisions they need to see the analytical financial data. Whether if its coaches, business owners or capitalist it is the measuring of progress by analyzing the numbers that will make the difference if you want to win. Consider yourself as the coach of your own body. If you want to play to win in losing weight, you will want to start tracking the numbers of what you're putting inside your body.

When you start to track the number of your daily calories you will gain a new perspective of what you are putting inside your body. If you want to gain the most effective results in the fastest amount of time it is best to keep a food journal and develop the habit of writing down everything you are consuming daily. Keep it within your reach wherever you go. Use a mobile app if you find that it's easier. There is no right or wrong way, just find what works for you.

By keeping a food journal and recording what you consume will allow your mind to see what you need to do to improve your total calorie intake for the day. The goal is to turn your day into a measurement of progress that contributes towards the step system of your weekly progress. By using the weekly step system and developing this habit will make it automatic. When you do this it will get to the point where you just do it without thinking about it and make it become part of your daily and weekly ritual. Keep this lifestyle change consistent and you are about to see some major changes happen after thirty days. Start getting at least 5 or 6 points a week using the weekly step system and when you look in the mirror thirty days from now you are going to like what you see. With these changes will come many compliments and positive feedback. This will result in you feeling better about yourself and the momentum of your progress will keep you going strong. Visualize this feeling. Learn to crave it and don't stop.

Write down what you are eating; use the weekly step system and play to win.

ACTION STEPS

1) Measure Your Progress - Break your progression down into a weekly measurement. Use the step system to measure and strive for a 6 out of 7 score for the week. Gain at least three successful weeks out of the month and you will be making progress and gaining momentum. Gain 4 successful weeks out of the month and you will be making serious progress and celebrating your quick results. When the mind has a clear measurement of how to achieve results it can then achieve results in a more focused and direct manner.

2) Practice Until It Becomes a Habit - Using the step system every day is practicing. Practice it until it becomes effortless and a lifestyle change.

3) Play to Win - Keep a food journal and track what you put inside your body. This awareness will change your health-conscious mindset.

CONCLUSION

Clarity to your goals is key. Use the Weekly Step System!

Chapter 4

Weight Loss Desires- What You Want

What do you think about on a consistently? If you are male, is it sex? Is it meeting with a hot date for this weekend or attending an important social event. Are you a family person that desires to go to the beach with your kids and have fun in the water? Regardless of who we are, it is the things that are taking place in our everyday lives that have a great deal of influence on the decisions we are making. However, it is our constant desires of what we think about that will mold our motivation.

For example, if you have an upcoming high school reunion soon on the horizon you will most likely want to be in the best shape possible to look your best. It is natural to want to appear as fit as possible since it has been a while since you have not seen many of your old friends. You may naturally begin to eat better and exercise vigorously. It's like a desire mechanism kicks in our minds and ignites a spark in some motivation gland in our brains. Is there a motivation gland? Why does this happen? The key to weight loss is desiring what you want consistently. When you do this it will help keep you in that same state of mind and give you the discipline that you need to stay motivated.

Desire what you want often. It's healthy for your weight loss motivation.

Feed That Mind With What You Want

The visualization process is the process of practicing what you desire and letting your thoughts turn you into the person you want to become. Becoming what we think about is a result of what we feed our minds with. This principle can be utilized to your advantage to train your mind to be a weight loss machine.

Example: If you wanted to become a chef or an expert at cooking you would need to learn about the many different attributes that make up a chef's talent. You would begin training your mind and learning cooking techniques. You may begin to watch YouTube videos on food preparation, read cookbooks, and revolving your thinking around your objective which is the simple desire to become what you think about.

The weight loss process uses this same principle. If want to become an expert in a certain field, feed your mind with everything it needs to know in that field.

The reason for this is you will harvest what you plant. If you planted seeds of Bermuda grass then you will get that type of grass and the same goes for any other plant.

Your desires are your seeds. Those desires may only be your thoughts in the beginning and not be physically tangible however when harvested and properly nurtured thoughts eventually transform into our world of physiology.

Our minds are fresh soil and weight loss is about desiring what you want so you can grow into the expert that you are capable of becoming. Plant your mind with the fitness knowledge it needs so that you can grow your fitness. Plant it with the healthiest, most positive information of healthy intellect that you want to grow it with.

Think about someone that comes to your mind that is very fit and in amazing shape. If you are male think of a male and female think of a female. Is the person that first comes to your mind an expert in the fitness field? Do you desire their body and wish your body looked more like theirs? Are they better, smarter, or more driven than you? Or did they simply decide to plant their minds with the thoughts that turned their bodies into a reality?

The answer is they fed their minds first. The truth is, you are enough. You are beautiful inside out and if you want to feel the same way on the outside then fill your mind with the beauty of fitness that you deserve to have.

It is difficult to get what you want if you don't feed that mind with the content it needs.

Imagine if you were going to fly a plane and have never done so in your life. Would it possible to pilot a plane without first learning the fundamentals, calibration of controls, and the meticulous details necessary to coordinate your flight path and reach your destination? Every single day dieters and overweight people overlook the process of becoming fit by choosing a different path to fly. They choose not to become experts and input the knowledge they need to become what they think about.

Decide to feed your mind with everything possible so that you can reach your fitness destination.

Use Vacations and Important Events to Motivate You

A cruise, marathon, wedding, or reunions are all samples of events that would motivate the amount of effort you put into fitness. For example, imagine if you told yourself that would like to lose 10 pounds by the 1st of next month versus you want to lose 10 pounds before you go on a cruise next month. You would be more motivated by the cruise.

It's about "our constant desires and what we think about" therefore utilize the way your brain works emotionally to your advantage.

We are thinking about the event constantly when faced with making daily decisions. These desires will tie in with the emotions of your motivation and is one of the most effective ways you can motivate yourself.

Your surroundings of people and choices to be involved in different events will ultimately affect what is on your mind. Use this to your advantage to motivate yourself. This gives you the upper hand to be savvy to maneuver through different events as part of your lifestyle in a direction that's motivated by your fitness goals. Make wise choices that get you involved with events that will stimulate your motivation so that your thoughts stay focused on exciting positive future events.

Try to view them as not only as times to support others but also as opportunities. These types of opportunities give you the ability to be in the most motivated state of mind possible. Plan your events well ahead of time to allow yourself to visualize how you want to look before your event. Emotional motivation is the most effective motivation therefore set your goals to control how you will emotionally motivate yourself. It is one of the most effective ways to control your actions.

"Our constant desires and what we think about are key elements to us making strides in our fitness goals."

Single People

Discomfort Levels Can Manifest Action

Single people naturally desire to be more attractive consistently more than non-single people.

If you are single you may think about sexual encounters more than the average married person. Your psychological needs start to become physical and the measures you may take to fulfill those needs may become more of a priority in your life. This level of discomfort generally manifests action without them realizing it and that many single people may not realize they are experiencing this discomfort unless it is something they have become accustomed to.

It does not mean that all single people desire to be more attractive than others. It just means that the majority of single people have a slight natural discomfort level without realizing it if they don't have partners. For many motivated singles that realize this it works to their advantage and many will strive to watch their figures naturally.

It is no different from the hungry entrepreneur that desires to be successful. Sometimes it is the financial struggle that motivates them. Discomfort can work to your advantage when it comes to your fitness health.

Non-Single People Have Higher Comfort Levels

People that are married or have a significant other are generally more comfortable. However, that does not mean they do not strive, wish, and dream to be more attractive, desirable, sexy, or physically fit any less than a single person does. There are a lot of married men and women that are in the circle of that desire and are striving to get themselves in that physically fit condition they used to be in before they met their spouse or significant other. "Comfort" plays a key part in getting them to the unhealthy state they may be in, however, they still desire to be fit just as much as a single person. When we feel good about ourselves we then, in turn, are better to others that are in our lives, therefore making the relationship stronger physically and emotionally.

We also want to be fit and healthy for our children so that we can participate more in their lives and be around longer to witness their lives. A married person or a person with a significant other has more reasons to get motivated than a single person. A single person will be doing it for two reasons. Find a partner and feel good about themselves.

A married person can be motivated by several reasons, to feel better about themselves, be more attracted to their spouse and vice versa. To have a sexual appetite that is exciting and plentiful with their spouse and make the relationship stronger with their spouse. If they have kids they can be motivated to be healthy for them as well.

What prevents the motivation for many? Self-worth.

Regardless of if a man or woman, some don't feel worthy, some do not have the self-esteem that it takes to say "hey, I need to take care of me first and then I can take care of you". How can we love others if we don't love ourselves? It's just like on a commercial airline when the flight attendants show you the procedure for low cabin pressure. You put the oxygen mask on yourself first, then the child.

This is the reason why people in relationships should be more motivated with a passion. Think about what is important to you and start stimulating your motivation gland.

You are enough and worth every reason to start loving yourself and start becoming physically fit right now. Love yourself, love strong to others and do it.

Love is strength.

ACTION STEPS

1) **Desire What You Want -** You become what you think about. Your actions will follow.

2) **Envision The Emotional Feelings -** It is so satisfying when you lose weight and then see someone from an event that has not seen you in a while compliment you. Take advantage of how our minds work emotionally to your advantage and use these events as opportunities to emotionally motivate your mind.

3) **Love Strong -** for you and others. You are enough, you can do it.

CONCLUSION

Realize what is important to you in life and make it a priority so that you can enjoy more of it. Longevity will thank you.

WORDS ARE POWERFUL - Helping others build confidence

Have you ever had a hard obstacle or a bully in your life that you needed to overcome?

A SECRET ABOUT ME IS WHEN I WAS IN THE 7TH GRADE I HAD A BULLY THAT PICKED ON ME... and not just a little I mean pretty bad...

I was a 12 yr old chubby kid and he would pinch my chest saying I had breast etc. all kinds of mean, hurtful things that I don't want to repeat. I don't want to mention his name here but it wouldn't surprise me if he's in prison by now. He was the new kid that came in from an island and all the kids (even 8th graders) were scared of him because he was so aggressive and would sometimes punch the lockers to make himself look tough. He used to pick on me when I would walk home from school and one day he broke my Xmas gift which was a Sega Game Gear (super awesome game machine at the time). I was heartbroken and he told me my nose was next 💀

I used to run home every day trying to avoid this bully and every time he saw me he would chase me and tell me that I better run fat boy. It was awful and this went on for a while. Nobody knew and I was so ashamed.

Until finally one day...

I'll never forget what a kid named Derek Anderson did and how he helped me. Derek was a kind-hearted stocky kid (for 7th grade) who played sports and got along with nearly all the kids. He saw I was troubled and asked me what was wrong. I told him. He said that I could take this kid who was a bully and I will never forget what he said...

"Gilbert, look how big you are.. look at your chest you look like you could bench press a lot." He asked other peers that were standing around, "hey check out Gilbert's chest, (tapping on me almost as if he was getting them to approve) doesn't it look like Gilbert can bench press a lot?" The other kids looked at me puzzled and slowly nodded, "yeah he looks strong." this gave me the confidence that I had been needing and all of a sudden I started to no longer feel like a helpless chubby kid and felt as though my weight was strength."

Derek said, "Let's go approach him and I will help you if something happens...let's go find him but I think you can take him". He said, "Meet me after school and we will find him."

Although afraid, suddenly I had some confidence and found the courage to listen to Derek.

I still remember like it was yesterday...

The after school bell rang and kids were leaving their classes getting ready to go home. It was outside under the hallway pavilion area and there were a lot of kids around watching. I remember Derek walking toward this bully and standing in front of him until he was just a few feet away. He stood there and stared at him. The bully knew Derek was looking at him but said nothing. Then, Derek sternly said...

Hey.. (he called him by his name) Do you have a problem with Gilbert?? I then slowly walked up to him so that I was standing in his clear view. It felt like slow motion. The bully looked over at me... I was scared to death had my fist clenched in my pockets but was ready .. I remember the bully looking into my eyes and he saw that I was no longer going to put up with his crap and ready to take him on if I had to. Then the bully kid paused... then shook his head no and walked away.

He never touched or bothered me again after that. I remember walking home from school and always looking over my shoulder to see if he was following me(even when I was by myself) but he never approached me again. He no longer saw me as an easy target, and I went on to become much happier in life. From that day forward any time I had an obstacle in my way I always felt that fire inside to ALWAYS stand up for myself.

I'm grateful for Derek. Even in the adult world your friends sometimes just need a little help. Even if its a stranger on the street, if you ever see someone that needs help HELP THEM. Don't be one of those people that are part of the bystander effect and do nothing! I am not talking about just physical bullies either.. maybe it's an abusive ex or verbally abusive coworker. Your friends might need guidance on how to handle them professionally and tactfully.

Or they may simply just need an ear to listen to show you care and that you stand behind them. Never forget how your small efforts and words can make a huge impact in someone else's life by standing behind them and giving them the confidence & encouragement they sometimes need to hear.

Are your friends or family pretty, smart, strong, funny, amazing, or pleasant to be around? Since life can be challenging sometimes we just need to hear the great things about ourselves or how we appear to others and this confidence boost can be all we need to reverse our limiting beliefs.

Thank you Derek. Even though I have not spoken to you in 25 yrs I still remember this like it was yesterday and I wanted to tell you THANKS for helping me.

-Gilbert

P.S. And for others reading this never hesitate to be that Derek in someone else's life if they need to hear your words because <u>*words are powerful*</u>*.*

Chapter 5

Shrinking Your Stomach Process

The stomach is a muscular organ that is very elastic in quality, thanks to a series of ridges along its interior surface wall called rugae. These expandable folds allow your stomach to expand and contract to meet the demands of your food intake. The size of the stomach, therefore, is variable and is not so much linked to your weight as to your eating habits. Shrinking your stomach is more mental than physical.

If you are a heavy eater it is essential to go through this mental process to be able to lose weight. This is the process of the stomach becoming accustomed to eating fewer calories throughout the day.

You may have seen the documentaries of extremely obese people consuming enormous amounts of food. Have you ever wondered if an individual is at an extreme obesity level ex: 500 pounds or more how are they able to eat so much food? Some extreme obese are capable of consuming 15 to 30 thousand calories in a single day, which is enough for the average person to eat in an entire week. This does not happen overnight.

It is developed over a period of time through a series of unhealthy habits of stretching the stomach to where it becomes large. When it's empty, the stomach is normally about the size of your closed fist. But because this organ has the ability to stretch, the more you eat, the more enlarged your stomach becomes to suit the volume of its contents. It shrinks back to its normal size through the natural course of digestion as food contents move out of the stomach and into the duodenum, and then on to the small intestine.

The good news is you can get your body used to eating fewer calories and feel satisfied without having surgery by gradually eating less.

This is also not done overnight and the same way is conditioning over a time period but if consistent you can do this without surgery on your stomach.

It's not possible to physically shrink the stomach beyond its normal size without surgery. It is, however, possible to feel full eating less food, which is generally the aim of wanting a smaller stomach. The way to accomplish this effect is to train your body to get used to accommodating smaller meals. Your stomach will adjust to proportions suitable for the needs of the average quantity of food you're used to taking in, in a single serving. Over time, eating smaller-portioned meals reduces the size your stomach is accustomed to inflating during mealtime.

When you consume food it takes approximately fifteen minutes for the initial food to settle in your stomach and the acids to begin breaking the solids down. Once this starts taking place the stomach can start registering the signals from the brain that it is full. The problem many people have is they do not give this process enough time to take place. They will generally eat more until it is already too late before the stomach has a chance to notify the brain with the message it is already satisfied.

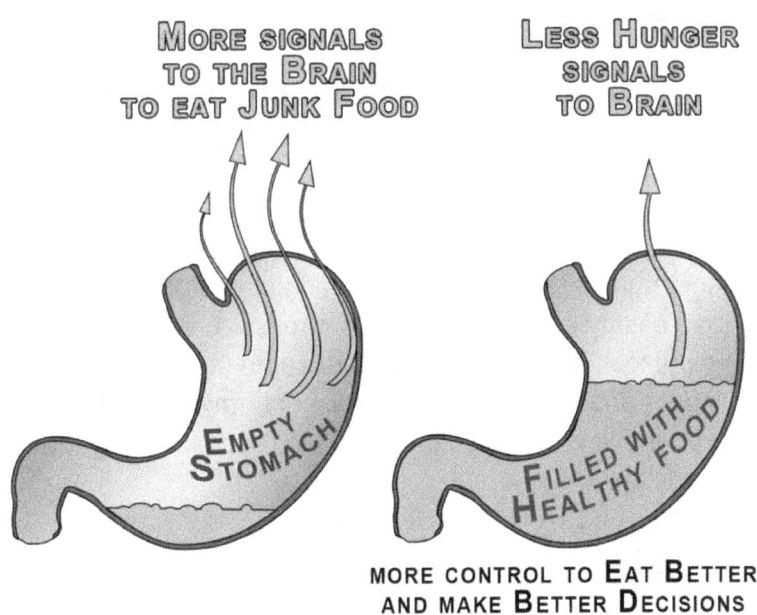

MORE SIGNALS
TO THE BRAIN
TO EAT JUNK FOOD

LESS HUNGER
SIGNALS
TO BRAIN

EMPTY STOMACH

FILLED WITH HEALTHY FOOD

MORE CONTROL TO EAT BETTER
AND MAKE BETTER DECISIONS

Dissatisfaction to Satisfaction

What determines if people lose weight or not is if they can get past the feeling of dissatisfaction to feel satisfyingly full. This satisfying feeling that you encounter once you have a full stomach is the comfort level that separates the individuals that make progress. It is the uncomfortable level that you must learn to deal initially while training your stomach. If you can get past this slight pain barrier you will succeed in your weight loss goals.

You must shrink your stomach and train your mind and body to have the capability to eat fewer calories to overcome the initial discomfort feeling. Think of the discomfort as the pain barrier you breakthrough. Arnold Schwarzenegger quoted this pain barrier as a type of obstruction during resistance training that would separate people who will succeed.

"If you can go through this pain barrier then you can succeed. If you can not go through this pain barrier then you will not succeed."

It kind of goes along with the saying no pain, no gain concept. Going through the shrinking the stomach process is an essential step to giving your mind and body, the weight loss abilities it needs to adapt to the fitness lifestyle. Understand this process and train your mind to start going through the barriers so that you can reach the body that you desire.

Eating For Necessity

When you get hungry you will eat food. This is a natural process of the body's survival mechanisms. It dates back to the cave days of how we live and survive. If we do not have this natural mechanism working for us we would not know when to eat to keep our bodies nourished. However, have you ever stopped to think about why we eat beyond this natural feeling of being satisfyingly full? These are the times of how we have evolved as people. We tend to eat beyond our comfort levels because the possibility for us to do so is easily accessible.

The act of eating beyond the requirements of necessity is simply out of pleasure. These are the times we eat because it is convenient. It satisfies the cravings of our taste buds and allows us to emotionally bond with others. Times have changed and eating for necessity is no longer the norm for most humans. By taking the step to read this you gain the understanding of eating for necessity and have the choice to enjoy the finer things life has to offer you.

When It Happened to You

If you are currently used to consuming more calories than you burn per day this was most likely a habit that was developed over time. You see somewhere along the lines of life you developed the habit that gradually turned into a daily regimen. It was probably done without you thinking about it or simply not focusing on the consequences of what would happen. For some of us, it happens during the comfort of marriage and for others, it happens early during childhood. It can happen to all types of people, single people, busy people, unemployed, depressed and even successful people. Anyone can fall into the trap of getting used to consuming more calories than they need daily. Although there is some benefit to understanding how it may have happened the most beneficial way to overcome it is to decide what you are going to do about it.

Drinking-Water

Much of the time that we think we are hungry we are simply dehydrated. Your body is craving water and much of the food we eat is made of water. This is a time for you to utilize drinking water to your advantage so that you can keep the hunger pains to a minimum. The next time you are feeling hungry don't suppress eating, just start by drinking water as an appetizer before you start digging into your next meal. It is healthier for digestion and has many other health benefits for your organs. When you go to an all you can eat buffet there is a reason why restaurants will keep your glass full. Just ensure you are drinking empty calories such as water. In the end, it will help you to feel more satisfied when you start eating your meal. Incorporate this technique combined with everything else you are learning here and it will help you with the stomach shrinking process.

Grocery Shopping With A Large Stomach

If you shop for groceries when you are hungry you are asking for trouble. Don't do it. It is one of the biggest mistakes you can make since it paves the foundations for your upcoming choices of foods. Every second that you are hungry, your mind is telling your body to eat. Making the best decisions starts at the grocery store, therefore this is the most important time you want to make sure your appetite is satisfied. Remember when you buy foods high in fat and sugar although they taste good this satisfaction is always temporary. The temporary satisfaction is always counterproductive to our overall health physically as well as mentally since having these foods in your house will bring extra stress to you by adding resistance to your mental strength against your goals. Shop with a smaller stomach. You will feel better in the long run as you start to feel better about your body.

ACTION STEPS

1) Have Awareness of The Discomfort That Will Pass - People that tend to become extremely obese may not identify why it is difficult for them to lose weight. Being conscious of the shrinking stomach process is crucial to your progress in cutting calories and eating less daily. Ensure yourself of the progress you are making as you deal with any discomfort levels while advancing your body to its weight loss capabilities.

2) Think About When You're Full - When finished eating a normal size meal take time out to pause and think about if you are full. By becoming attentive to the fullness sensation you are taking a step towards the shrinking of your stomach process.

3) Develop The New Habit of Feeling Satisfied - Recognize the fact that your eating habits developed sometime in your earlier life and were developed over time. Just as any habit is developed over time it takes time to break the habit. Develop a new habit to never eat to where you feel overly stuffed.

CONCLUSION

When you train your body to become accustomed to eating smaller meals you lay a foundation of future dieting success by giving your body new capabilities. It's like an old sports car going to 60mph faster. Sometimes we just need a tune-up.

THOUGHT OF DYING - Scared To Sleep

It's the middle of the night around 3:00 AM and I am awoken from sleep by a severe burning sensation in my throat and chest.

It's so bad that I feel as if I am having a heart attack. One particular time the pain was so unbearable that I thought I was dying and did not know what to do.

I rushed to the refrigerator to drink something cold out of desperation and began drinking tea straight from the container. What I didn't know was that I was having extreme heartburn. It was a result of being obese and it was affecting me every single night but that night it was the worst than it had ever been. I didn't know what to do and waited for the cold tea to numb my pain but it didn't.

I yelled loudly with a deep grunt as if I was gasping for air. The pain was unbearable and I kept grunt yelling. It seemed like the pain was getting worse and the cold tea was not helping.

What I did not know was that the caffeine in the tea was a stimulant that amplifies acid reflux. It made the pain worse. I did not sleep that night and the next day I could feel the soreness in my esophagus for days.

This traumatic event made me realize that I was obese. It's easy to get caught up in the mindset that, as long as you're happy, it is okay if you are overweight. I wasn't happy with this pain, feeling like I was dying in the middle of the night. I didn't know if I was having a heart attack or what was happening. I wasn't happy and I didn't want to be overweight.

This event influenced my decision to change my life and start living differently.

Chapter 6

In the Zone

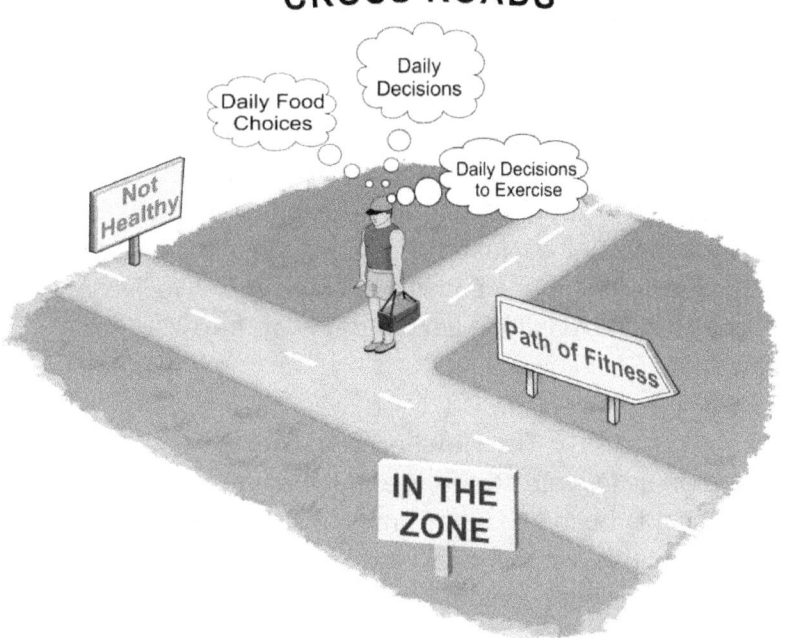

Being in the zone is where you want to be. It is the state of being extremely motivated. This is the state of your mind being so focused that your actions constantly reflect positive reinforcements to move you towards your weight loss objectives.

This is where you visualize your goals and how you want your body to look every time you come to the crossroads of a decision. People that are into fitness generally live in the zone without much effort since it is what they are used to. Most of us do not stay in this zone of motivation. This is not necessarily your fault. As you read this if you do not live in the zone it is your decision and responsibility to make that directional choice. Not being in the zone is more common because of the many conditions of the world we live in today that have influenced our paths we travel.

The Howling Dog Story

One of my favorite stories is about the nail and the howling dog. It has been told many times to show the analogy of pain and how we relate to it if we take action. It's about getting out of the content comfort zone so you can be comfortable in the end.

There was once a young boy who was walking to school. On his way to school, he passed the house of an old man who was sitting on his front porch with an old dog sitting next to him howling away. "How weird", he thought to himself.

On the way home, he passed the same house of the old man and the dog was still sitting on the porch howling. Again the young boy thought to himself that this was rather strange.

This same scene, of the old man and howling dog, repeated itself for two days before the young boy finally built up the courage to inquire of the old man exactly why his dog was sitting on the porch and howling every day. The young boy approached the old man and asked, "Why is it that every time I come across your house your dog just sits there howling? Is there something wrong with him?" The old man looks at the boy and responds, "Nope. There's nothing wrong with him. The idiot sat on a nail a few days ago and it hurts him like hell." Completely confused, the boy asks, "Well, then, why doesn't he just get up off that nail?" The old man quickly replies, "I guess it doesn't hurt him bad enough."

Sometimes in life, we have many nails that are always poking at us. You may have things that bother you whether in your career, personal life, or your body. Sometimes it will hurt enough for you to just yowl about it once in a while. Other times the pain may be so bad that it causes you to take action and move on it. Every action we take in life is generally one of two things. It is either to move towards a sense of pleasure or avoid a sense of pain.

The howling dog story gives us a clear vision of how we can view our actions. Decide if the nail is hurting you bad enough. Then decide if you want to take your mind into the zone.

Bad Programming

Sometimes some things work against us. For example, one of the abundant influencing factors is preprogramming.

Not being in the zone can simply be a result of bad programming.

We have experienced this growing up. Everywhere around us, advertisements are telling us to eat bad quality foods. Studies show that it takes an average of seven times for the brain to register the product in the subconscious mind as a permanent memory. By seeing fast food and juicy steak house ads day by day, year after year, the programming in the average person's mind is filled with subconscious thoughts they are not aware of. When we have the opportunity to eat healthy foods versus unhealthy foods our minds have been pre-programmed with thoughts to our disadvantage. How many advertisements have you seen that promotes you to eat healthy foods rather than unhealthy? The unhealthy ads dominate the ad market since the natural cravings of consumers result in higher profitability to unhealthy food distributors and manufacturers.

Win The Battle

This is the reason it is imperative to start training the brain to battle our conditions around us. The unhealthy food messages are capitalizing and killing us every day without us realizing it. The reason nearly 60% of Americans are overweight is due to bad programming. To deal with the issue to win the war in improving our nation's unhealthy state, we must be able to recognize the problem. Every billboard ad, fast food commercial, or advertisement that influences us to make bad decisions must be an opportunity to turn it into a good thought at the crossroads to be in the zone. Every time you see an ad for unhealthy food try to think of something healthy to supplement it. If you see a hamburger commercial try to envision a healthy dish that you enjoy. Beat the food corporations and extensiveness of life and happiness will thank you.

Our New World

We have become used to things as human beings to include routines and regimens. Routine for us has become a world of effortless food sources and a decrease in physical activities such as escalators, moving sidewalks in airports, and advanced technology that allows us to decrease our activity level. Nowadays our physical activities have evolved to more leisure and recreational whereas before physical activities were out of necessity. This means that our world is evolving into a more effortless one and the decision to go into the health zone is more of a decision that is our individual choice.

How We Adapt

What our bodies are used to is a result of the conditioning that we have made possible. For example: Imagine the old west days before modern inventions such as cars and air conditioning. Air conditioning is an example of our minds and bodies being used to what we know. In fact, the very part of the meaning of the word illustrates just that point "conditioning". Back in the old days, it was not necessarily uncomfortable for people to not have air conditioning because they never had it. In our present world if a person lives in the south in the heat of the summer they must get to a cool shelter or they may risk overheating. This is an example of "How we adapt".

We as people today are used to the many things in our everyday lives that condition our minds and bodies to be unhealthy. For example when the mind is familiar with something it goes into a comfort zone. Imagine the smell of a person in the old west days before air conditioning and also the invention of deodorant. What kind of scent did the average man give off? Most farm animals when in the slightest proximity give off a distinct natural smell. At one time humans had their own strong musky smell that signified our nature before the invention of deodorant, however, it was not a problem to us in those days. Nowadays let an average adult go without the invention of deodorant for just a couple days and the musky smell would be unacceptable compared to today's standards. This is a result of what our minds have become used to in our comfort zone. Our world today is filled with things that have conditioned us to be comfortable while making us unhealthy and we don't even think about it. Try to break away from the world's conditions that work against your health and fitness. Try to condition yourself to be in a healthy state by breaking away from what you are familiar with such as all the bad programming and limited physical activity. Try to enter into the zone using the power of your mind to overcome all your conditions around you.

Acceptance

For some people, they may not be in the zone for the simple fact of acceptance. This is where we as people have accepted what is taking place in our everyday lives and have accepted our level of comfort. You do not have to do this. You do not have to settle and owe it to yourself to be the very best that you want to be. Do not settle and go into the fitness zone.

ACTION STEPS

1) Make Decisions at the Crossroads - Every single day, every decision you make is at the crossroads. Plant your mind with these thoughts and you will set yourself up to influence yourself internally to make the right decisions.

2) Overcome the World's Conditioning - Realize and understand the conditions that work against you, however, do not focus on them. Be conscious of how most people fall into the traps and adapt to the world's conditioning. Once you have grasped the concept of how to work against the entire negative input you can fight back and win.

CONCLUSION

Studies have shown that environments influence how people arise. You have been put into an environment of today's world. It is up to you to choose how you will arise.

"The choice is yours if you will adapt to what most have adapted to or beat the resistance and achieve your dreams."

Chapter 7

Super Weight Loss Focus

Focus Abilities

Brain Clutter

Brain clutter is everywhere. It distracts your focus from accomplishing your goals. Think of clutter as noise. If you are trying to listen closely to something and there is a lot of noise around it makes it difficult to focus on listening. People tend to forget that all the brain clutter in their life makes it hard for them to achieve their goals. If this is an obstacle you are faced with, it's okay because you can quickly and easily resolve this.

The first step to eliminating brain clutter is understanding the importance of how it affects you so you understand how to resolve it.

Think of a vehicle that is running hard in the hot sun with the air conditioner on full blast. A combustion engine must run hard to regulate the vehicle's cooling system. If you shut the a/c totally off sometimes you may notice a slight amount of increased horsepower in the vehicle.

National Geographic did a study on the brain's ability to focus. They were able to determine that everything in your peripheral vision, from the sounds you hear, to the movements you are doing, to what you mind is thinking about all makes a difference in how hard your mind is working.

Have you ever sat in front of a messy desk? Your mind may be thinking about all the things you need to do from one pile to the next rather than getting things done. Studies show that you can be more effective if you focus on one thing at a time.

Organize yourself so you can set yourself up for weight loss performance. For example, if you were a baker and wanted to specialize in cakes, you would need to become an expert in cake baking. To be most effective, you would need to remodel your kitchen to be equipped with commercial grade appliances, baking goods at your fingertips, as well as schooling/education specifically in baking cakes. For your super weight loss focus mindset, you will need to have healthy foods at your fingertips and information/cookbooks with healthy recipes. Start by organizing your kitchens health arsenal and remember if you don't buy it you won't eat it so start organizing and setting yourself up for easier success.

Your stress level depends on the amount of brain clutter in your life. Work on eliminating all the extra distractions in your life that do not contribute to your new focused in the zone mindset and your mind will run effectively and fire clean on all cylinders.

Don't worry if it seems too overwhelming.

For example when you do laundry and dump a basket full of socks on a bed that needs to be paired. The laundry clutter is everywhere and seems like it will take forever. The sooner you start to pair which sock goes with its matching pair you put each of the paired up socks to the side. The more socks you pair the easier it becomes to pair the rest of the load with every new two socks you pair up and it continues to become easier and faster. Cleaning up your life's brain clutter is no different. As the saying goes, "How do you eat an elephant?" One bite at a time, so the sooner you get started the easier it will get.

Losing a large amount of weight is a very similar process. If you have a large amount of weight to lose do not feel discouraged. Looking at the long road ahead of you appears harder than it really is because once you begin it starts to immediately become easier. Becoming used to new foods, new exercise routines, and a healthy lifestyle may appear like a lot in the initial phase. However, just as mentioned above it is the same as pairing socks. The sooner you begin, the easier it starts to get. Once you start, within about one to two weeks you will begin to notice how much easier it becomes. After thirty days you will notice the focus that it took in the initial phase to get started becomes effortless. Since new habits can develop over a thirty-day time period this is all the time you need to gain your new super weight loss focus.

Filtering out all of life's distractions is important for weight loss and is overlooked in the fitness world. Give your life balance and you will give your life clarity to lose weight.

"One does not accumulate but eliminate. It is not daily increase but daily decrease. The height of cultivation always runs to simplicity." – Bruce Lee

Active Brain

If you grew up in the 80's you may remember an anti-drug commercial used to illustrate what drugs do to your brain with just three phrases. The commercial shows hot butter cooking in a skillet with the narrator saying "This is drugs" followed by the cracking of an egg onto the hot skillet, with the narrator saying "This is your brain on drugs." As the egg immediately begins sizzling, the narrator, "Any questions?"

With exercise, this is the exact opposite. If more people understood the effect exercise has on their brains we would have more of an active population. We need a commercial that illustrates the positive effects to show how exercise stimulates our mental activity.

Below is an image that shows what the brain looks like when it's on exercise.

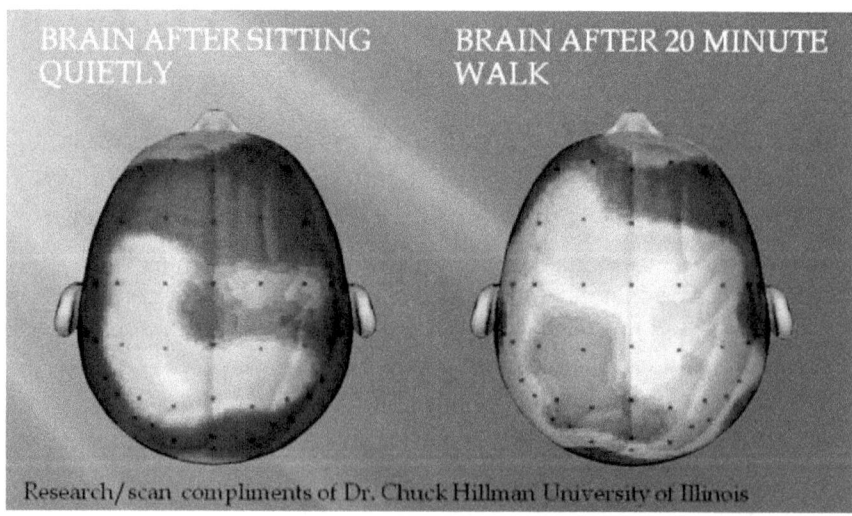

Research/scan compliments of Dr. Chuck Hillman University of Illinois

By viewing this illustration should bring awareness of why many successful entrepreneurs and active people are energetic and innovative. This is one of the reasons why many highly active people cannot seem to stop coming up with their genius ideas and why they may excel at many tasks. When you are focused on an active lifestyle of fitness this helps contribute towards putting you into overall alignment. The more you exercise the more you will be focused. The more you are focused the more you will be in alignment to exercise more and the momentum continues.

Imagine the chocolate topping syrup that becomes a hard shell after you place it on ice cream. They sell this at the grocery store and if it has been sitting in your cabinet for a while the sediments will settle and like many food products they must be shaken before use. If not it doesn't work as effectively. This is the same with many medicines and other products that have a liquid form. Shaking them helps them taste better, work effectively and revives their potency. If you are always sitting on the couch your blood is not pumping throughout your body as well as your brain and you will be settled. This is why it's important to go for a walk if you have been sitting for too long. Just as the above illustration shows how the brain is more active you must get the blood flowing through your head to revitalize the different parts of your brain waking up the neurons so they can receive the maximum amount of oxygen.

Don't let the blood in your brain be settled and get it flowing every day revitalizing its maximum potency so your focus can be at its prime. Exercise has many benefits to the brain as shown below.

YOUR BRAIN ON EXERCISE

Access Your Body's Own Legal Pharmacy Resources

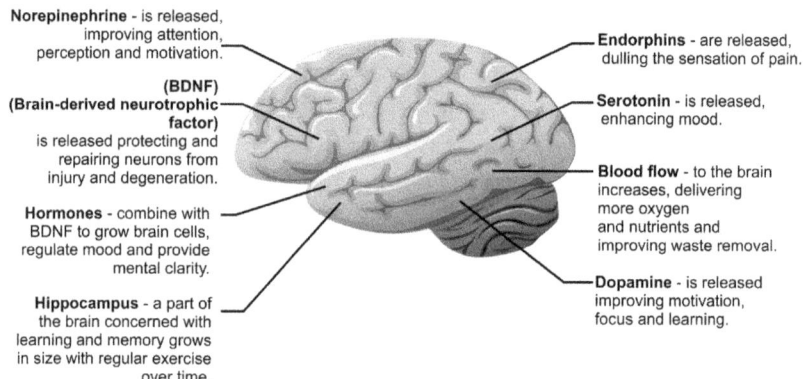

Norepinephrine - is released, improving attention, perception and motivation.

(BDNF)
(Brain-derived neurotrophic factor) is released protecting and repairing neurons from injury and degeneration.

Hormones - combine with BDNF to grow brain cells, regulate mood and provide mental clarity.

Hippocampus - a part of the brain concerned with learning and memory grows in size with regular exercise over time.

Endorphins - are released, dulling the sensation of pain.

Serotonin - is released, enhancing mood.

Blood flow - to the brain increases, delivering more oxygen and nutrients and improving waste removal.

Dopamine - is released improving motivation, focus and learning.

Many people overlook the benefit of exercising to gain mental clarity and the ability for the brain to think at its prime is overlooked by many as a benefit to exercising. It's not only the body that needs exercise but also the mind. Start taking decisive action to exercise so you have an active brain as well as an active body to contribute to your weight loss focus.

Weight Loss Time Is Investing

Our focus time towards weight loss is a huge investment.

Envision time as a daily deposit. You receive this daily deposit of time every day and regardless it gets spent at the end of each day on whatever you choose. We are also allowed to spend the amount of time we wish on our fitness goals and health.

Thinking with this mindset imagine for example if you were given $100 per day to spend on fitness and the dollars were equivalent to minutes. How much would you spend on fitness? Most people say they don't have the time to spend. However, overall this is very counterproductive to your life.

When you do not invest the amount of time every day on your health your daily deposit can stop immediately because your lifespan can get shortened by 20, 30 or even 50 years. Do you truly believe you do not have the time to spend on your health or is it not a priority? Remember our investment of time is being spent every day regardless of our decisions. Invest in you. Invest the time now so your investment can grow.

Longevity will allow you to be there for your family as long as possible. Your daily deposit is limited and goes away every day so ensure to spend it wisely and spend some of it on fitness every single day for you to receive your return on your investment.

You.

Your Work Vs Time For Fitness

Your focus abilities allow you to focus more on fitness. This is why this chapter is essential because it is this focus bandwidth that must be freed up to help you bring balance in your life.

"The time it took you to gain the weight versus the time it takes you to lose it is your decision."
Generally, people that become very motivated who are not used to a change in lifestyle go into a shock of changing their health habits. It may be a total makeover in routine for

them to be waking up to go to the gym in the mornings and eating healthy.

"I don't have time to work out" vs "I don't have time to brush my teeth"

Is taking care of your body a part of your lifestyle that you don't necessarily think or struggle about doing or do you just do it?

Some people might say I don't have time to work out, however, generally, they will not say I don't have time to brush my teeth or do something essential in their life. Although some people have more of an ability to focus on health because they have more time on their hands or a less stressful life but in the end, we all face the same health decisions. However, regardless we are all still given the same amount of time to spend every day. How we spend it is up to us. The time to spend it on your health is now!

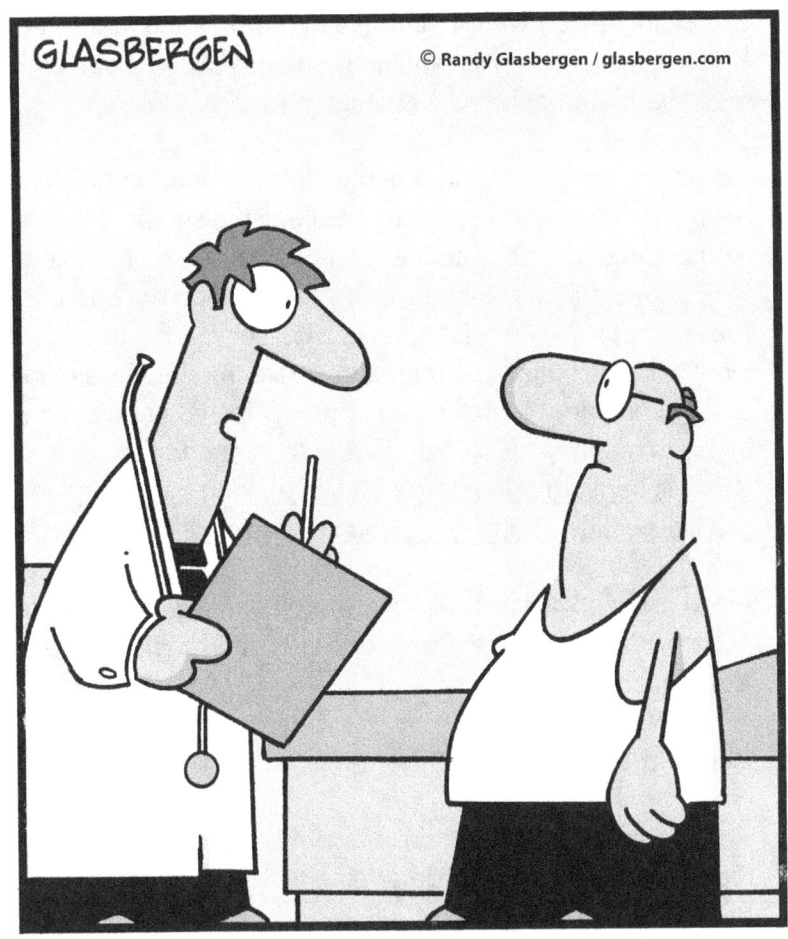

"What fits your busy schedule better, exercising one hour a day or being dead 24 hours a day?"

Exercise - Life or Death?

Hypothetically speaking, pretend you are given a choice and had to choose only one maintenance upkeep for yourself to maintain your health. Imagine if you were given the choice to choose between brushing your teeth or exercising. If you were to choose exercising and you never brushed your teeth you would end up having very bad breath and probably not a pleasant smile.

However, if you chose to brush your teeth and to never exercise most likely your body would diminish and your life would end earlier than usual. You see people do not seem to realize the importance of exercise. They do not seem to realize that if they do not keep bodies active they are slowly diminishing to an unhealthy state and they are dying earlier compared to active fit people. Once you realize the logistics of this you will understand the importance. You will begin to understand that by making the choice to live life healthy is simply making the choice to live longer.

If you are motivated to reach your goals make exercising a priority in your life so that this decision stays inside your focus bandwidth.

Best Time for Activity Time

The times you decide to make activity or gym time your focus during the day will determine the outcome of your best results.

Many experts will debate which times are best for the body to exercise. Some may insist that later in the day when your muscles are warm and strength may be at it's highest is best. Some may say when your energy level is high in the morning is better for cardio. The best time to exercise is the best time it will ensure you get it done. Once you become accustomed to the activity of having an exercise routine then fit it in your schedule that is most effective to ensure you complete your activity time. If you are flexible and must select a time based on the studies of science then experts will generally recommend morning times are the most effective times when your energy level is full. Remember as the day goes by so does your energy, so make sure not to wait too late. If you continue to put off exercising throughout the day the very thought of constantly thinking about exercising itself will drain you. Rather than procrastinate just get it out of the way and get it done. Once it is done you will have the reward of accomplishment and a task that is off your to-do-list. This will then have a psychological effect on how you eat and the decisions you make for more progress throughout your day.

Find the time for your activity time; the best time is your time.

Calorie Deficit Choice

It is necessary to go into a calorie deficit daily if you are going to make progress on losing weight. This is the state the body must be in consistently where you are burning more calories a day than you are consuming. If you are overweight you did not get to be overweight in one night. The excess weight was gained over a period of time. "The key to losing body fat is the simple decision if you choose to be in a daily calorie deficit and how many times per week you decide to do it."

Adjusting Focus Over Time

If you have just started a new diet and exercise program as a beginner practicing this discipline for only three days may feel like forever. For someone that is not used to being in a calorie deficit on a daily basis, this may be a shock to their body and challenge their mental comfort. You need to confront this shocking period and understand the time it is going to take before it becomes easier. Realize it is all about mental comfort. This shock at first may make you uncomfortable to be in a calorie deficit especially if it is something that you have never experienced. Through conditioning, what is uncomfortable today can become comfortable in the future. As a beginner having this temporary discomfort, in the beginning, is totally normal. Imagine running several miles you were not used to running or climbing a mountain you have never climbed. Your mind and body will be affected by the simple fact that it has never done it before. Just as the pool water can become warm after submerging yourself for a period of time, your comfort level will begin to adjust. This is the same when adjusting your focus to be in a calorie deficit. Your body will eventually adjust to comfort.

Complete a task often and as time passes by so would the activity of doing it without us even thinking about it. This is the comfort level you need to reach. This is the adjustment that needs to happen over a period of time. The reason many people fail at dieting and exercise is they get to the discomfort level in the beginning stage and automatically assume that their fitness quest is always going to feel uncomfortable developing a false belief that it is always hard. They are misled by assuming that there will always be discomfort feelings causing many to quit early. Now that you have a clear understanding of the focus that will be required to get through the discomfort period, take your time. Take a deep breath and submerge yourself in the pool water and let the discomfort pass so you can get into the zone of comfort.

Give it time and before you know it you will be in a comfortable calorie deficit on a daily basis feeling great every day losing all the weight you want.

ACTION STEPS:

1) Time Makes The Focus Easier - Just as the pairing of socks gets easier as you put away laundry is similar when you begin to remove the brain clutter in your life. The more balance you get, the easier it gets to lose weight.

2) Remember to Keep an Active Brain - Stay active with exercise and the more you do the better focused you will be. Exercising will help you keep an active brain, which will keep you in alignment to continue the momentum to stay focused.

3) Do not waste your daily deposit of time - Spend some of it on fitness and think of it as an investment to spend more time with your loved ones. In the business world, this is referred to as ROI (Return On Investment). The ROI on fitness is extremely high therefore in Motivational Weight Loss this is your ROL (Return On Life).

4) Recognize the time is now - Start eating right, start exercising, and start adapting. Spend your time wisely. Get into a calorie deficit and understand the longer you do it the easier it gets.

CONCLUSION

By choosing the opportunity to focus on being healthy is

simply choosing the opportunity to live longer.

IGNORE THE DISTRACTIONS - Pull yourself up

When I was a chubby kid in school I remember trying to do pull-ups for a P.E. test.

A bunch of the skinny kids watching laughed at me because our coach Ms. Hallway (she was awesome to me) had to hold my feet while I tried to pull myself up.

She had her clipboard in one hand and with the other, she tried to lift my shoes and said, "Pull!" as she told those kids, "Don't laugh at him!"

I tried so hard but couldn't do it 💀.

And they still laughed.

I remember her whispering to me, "Ignore them Gilbert."

Many years later I never forgot that whisper.

Any time something is not going right and I think people are laughing at me I remember that voice.

And now...

These days even at age 41, I can pull myself up 😌

We can get better with age! The words you speak create the world around you.

Feeling grateful. Age graceful.

Maintain your focus and ignore the distractions.

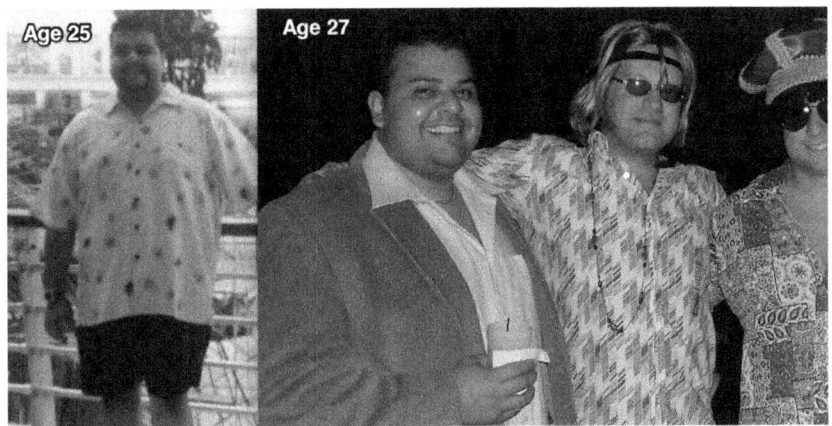

I let myself balloon to nearly 300lbs by the time I reached 27
and I was obese throughout my entire twenties.

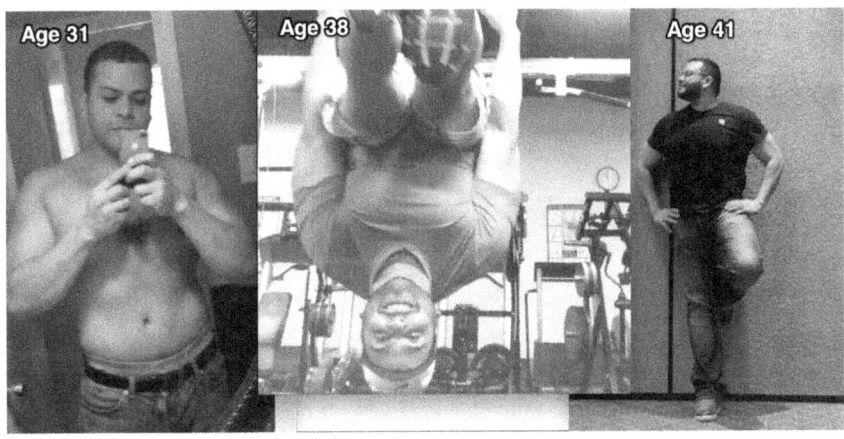

Although not perfect, I've been very grateful to live much
healthier in my older years.

Chapter 8

The Right Partner

There's a saying for success. It is to look at the 5 closest friends in your life and in 5 years your life will consist of the average of these 5 individuals. Why is that? It is because habits are contagious. It has much to do with mimicking our culture and environment obviously without us even realizing it. Now whether we realize it or not, did you know the person you decide to have as your partner in life will have the most direct impact on the lifestyle you live? Do you think its accident that obese children many times have overweight parents? It is no secret that who we let in our lives will influence our behaviors without us realizing it. There's a saying that you should not look at a person's physical appearance rather you should appreciate people for who they are on the inside. This is absolutely true. Although this is a good rule to live by, also realize that the partners you choose in life will most likely affect your overall health as well.

They are either supportive of your health-conscious decisions and will either encourage you or give you resistance. If you have made the decision to live a healthy lifestyle and currently have or plan to have a partner relationship then there are some key factors to remember. They are either "with you" (supportive of your decision), "against you" (not supportive and give you resistance) or "joining you" (teaming up with you on your plan).

1) "With You" Supports Your Decision - In the beginning, talk with your partner on your decision to change your lifestyle. Discuss expectations of things they can do to help support you. Discuss changes and things they can do on their part that will be mutually respectful of your health-conscious lifestyle so that it helps them be supportive of your decision to live healthy.

2) "Against" Gives You Resistance - Hopefully this is not your case and I hope that you currently have a supportive partner. In the event you do not, I would advise you to talk to your partner to see how you can get them to be supportive. Generally, there is usually a reason for someone to want to disapprove of their partner's decision to live healthy. It could be insecurities, selfishness, or some other reason that's bothering them. Communication is key and it's important to talk with your partner to see what is bothering them to not want to support you. In the end, it would not be morally ethical for someone else to not want you to live a long prosperous healthy life and in the event, your partner is still not supportive then you should consider seeking professional counseling. If a partner is still unsupportive of you wanting to change your life to live a healthy lifestyle then you should consider evaluating if it is in the best interest to stay in your relationship.

or

3) "Joining You" Do It Together - Discuss how you can work together to have a positive impact for both of you so that it reinforces your health and fitness through encouragement and support for each other. When both of you decide to live a healthy lifestyle you will be able to participate and agree on terms to support each other. This mutual decision creates momentum so you both can work together towards a common goal.

Our partner will have an influence on our decisions on a daily basis since we tend to mimic other's habits without really realizing we are doing it. We may not necessarily want to mimic them however sometimes it just affects our subconscious mind naturally. Whether it's your spouse, boyfriend, best friends, etc. They generally make up a part of our identity of the kind of people we are. Since the person we choose to spend the most time with effects our lifestyle choose them wisely. If you have already chosen your partner then try to accomplish 1 or 3 above this paragraph.

If you have not chosen your lifetime partner yet or are indecisive of a potential future relationship then ask yourself these basic questions.

1) How motivated is your partner?
2) Is fitness a priority to them?
3) If not, is it possible for fitness to become a priority in their lives?
4) If not, is it possible for them to be supportive of your fitness decision as a priority in your life?

This is an important step since your partner will have a dramatic influence on how they impact your life. The driving force of momentum can quickly turn if you can get the support of your partner to either help, push or join you.

If You Don't Buy It, You Won't Eat It.

The dinners that you make and eat together will now impact your relationship if only one person has changed their lifestyle. If one is motivated to live a fitness lifestyle and the other is not then the person that is not motivated will create temptation for the other. Unfortunately, this creates resistance for the relationship, which is the reason why you generally see fit couples paired with each other as well with unfit couples.

If you are in a situation with someone who constantly brings junk food into the household will you be motivated enough to resist the constant cravings? It will depend if the motivated partner is disciplined enough to overcome the temptations. Many have this discipline and for some, they can stay on track regardless of what foods are in front of them. However for someone who is not used to a fitness lifestyle of making the right choice it will be more difficult for them to deal with the constant temptation. It is recommended that they talk to their partner to either support them in their fitness goals or join them in the fitness lifestyle. Either way, it is imperative to address so that both partners can achieve happiness and reach fitness success together.

Imagine a person that is trying to stop smoking only to come home and see their partner smoking. This will put the person that is trying to quit in a more challenging situation because of the temptation that is always in the house. This works the same for bad food craving temptations. This is the reason why it is so beneficial to have a partner that supports you. It is even more beneficial if they can join you because their buying decisions can have an impact on your progress.

If you take the time to learn how to communicate with your partner to join your efforts it will make it much easier for both of you.

Example:

"Hey sweetie, I want us to live a long and healthy life together. It is important to me that I can get your support for us to live healthy. Will you help me so we can work as a team and we do this together?"

Divorce rates are at an all-time high because many people do not take the time to learn how to communicate effectively in a healthy manner. When we communicate properly we can do it in a fashion that rather creating friction, it instead ignites a desire in our partner to want to help and support us. Love and support each other starting now. Live happy and healthy together.

He or she wants to spend time with you.

The need to feel loved and our social surroundings are a normal part of our lives. If you are in a relationship you may find that this plays a huge factor in the daily decisions you make depending on if your partner is living a fitness lifestyle. Since our partners will generally want our time spent with them this will many times determine if we go to the gym or influence if we eat a healthy dinner. This will also depend on what level of motivation our partners are in their own lives. Talk to your partner. Let them know how important fitness is to you and what you would like to change. The most beautiful moments can be when our loved ones share the same passions with us and achieve goals together to strengthen our relationships.

ACTION STEP:

1) Check if Your Partner Will Support Your Fitness

Goals - The right partner could likely be the person you are with since they have chosen you in their life as well. Ask if they will support your goals. If they have chosen the path to be with you then most likely they will choose the next path to support your decision to change your life.

2) Sign Them Up With You - When you are aware of how mirroring habit alters people you will be aware of how much your partner makes the difference. Since a healthy lifestyle change is so dramatic having your partner's support will help you. Get them on board any way you can or better yet, get them to join you. Have them read this book as well.

CONCLUSION

Two heads are better than one generally speaking. Ideas, innovation, techniques, and synergy can come from building off each other's energy. This strength and bonding is like nothing else and is indescribable. Help stimulate each other's mind so that you both can reach your fitness destinations and achieve your returns of investment on life together.

PASSING THE TORCH - Big Dave

If you ever encounter someone such as a friend that is into fitness and are willing to train with you consider yourself very lucky and take them up on the opportunity.

Many people take fit friends for granted because personal trainers can be costly.

If a friend ever offers to workout with you and you think

they would be a positive influence, then do it.

When I was in my twenties I let myself balloon up to nearly 300lbs.

I knew how to work out but it was mainly from reading muscle magazines in the 90's when I was a teenager. I never really had anyone to actually "train me" and show me how to do exercises correctly.

I started my weight loss journey in 2007 at age 29. Initially, I was able to drop around 25 lbs from going on walks and working out in my garage from remembering what I read in the muscle magazines.

Even though I started losing weight I still needed that extra push to go to the next level because I started to slightly plateau on my weight loss.

In the beginning, I was too ashamed to start going to the gym because I was worried about what people would think.

I remember I had a good friend named Dave that was into fitness. Dave was around 47 at the time. He was from the Philippines but looked more Samoan because of his height and very muscular build. He previously competed in bodybuilding competitions in his younger years but even though he was older he still maintained his muscularity.

He would wear golf shirts and his arms would fill the sleeves. Dave owned a carpet cleaning business and he could always be seen driving his work vans, walking around town full of energy and always staying busy.

He offered to train with me and work out together. He said let's work out! Meet me at 6:15 AM.

I remember thinking, I'm usually still sleeping at that time but something told me to take him up on the opportunity. I thought, why not 6:00 AM or 6:30 AM? It was like he put thought into the exact time to make it physiological. 6:15 AM sharp it was!

I met him in a shopping center gym called Cove Fitness. Dave knew the gym owner Paul and I didn't even have a membership yet. Dave said "don't worry, you are with me. Let's get to working out and you can become a member later."

We immediately jumped into an ab workout routine. We started doing leg lifts, concentrated half crunches, side obliques and would alternate.

By the time I was done with the ab work out I was already out of breath and tired. Dave said, "okay now we are warmed up!"

I remember thinking... if this was the warm-up how am I going to be able to get through this work out because I was already out of breath?

But I did. We trained and did different workouts. Back, chest, legs.

Every day when we were done, he would point me to the cardio machines and say, "now make sure you do at least 20 to 30 minutes of cardio." He would then go to work and I would finish my work out.

After about 3 to 4 months of this routine, I started seeing results. I was always there, on time. One day he was running late and he said, "I'll be there, just get started."

It was odd not having him at first but I got started.

Shortly after that, he began missing a few days and when he did, he would work out in the afternoon.

At first, I was puzzled. I remember working out by myself wondering if he would make it for a few days in the morning.

The next time I saw him I asked him, "Hey, what happened? I thought we were going to keep working out?"

He looked at me with a look of frustration accompanied by a half-grin and he said, "if I'm not there, just work out." "You got this" as he nodded yes, "Just work out."

I realized at that moment that this was him passing the torch. Empowering me to be independent and do workouts on my own.

I went on to working out by myself, training myself and disciplining myself to stick with workouts based on everything I learned from Dave. Occasionally I would work out with friends or different partners but in the end, if they quit, I stuck with my routine and did not let my fitness health depend on anybody else but me.

When you begin your routine... whether if it's with a partner or not, friend, family member, relationship, or a trainer. There is one thing that needs to ultimately happen.

You are going to come to a time of realization.

Nobody is coming to save you. It is up to you.

Whether if you are fortunate enough to have a work out partner in the beginning or not.

You will come to a place of realization.

And when this happens... it means it's time to take the initiative. Time to take action for yourself.

And when that torch is passed to you... make sure you help someone else later on.

And empower someone else.

Because the right partner, is empowered in all of us.

Chapter 9

Your Social Events

When it comes to losing weight and maintaining fitness one of the most difficult obstacles to hurdle over are social events. This is where much weight is gained and where many fall off track. The amount of social events you attend on a regular basis makes the difference here. Your social event can be your cheat time to splurge and enjoy yourself if it is a rare occasion. If you are the type of person that hosts or attends numerous gatherings and entertains often then you will want to make sure you read this chapter closely for the mental preparation you will need. The social event is broken down into four fundamental obstacles that you must understand to be able to hurdle over them.

1) Alcohol

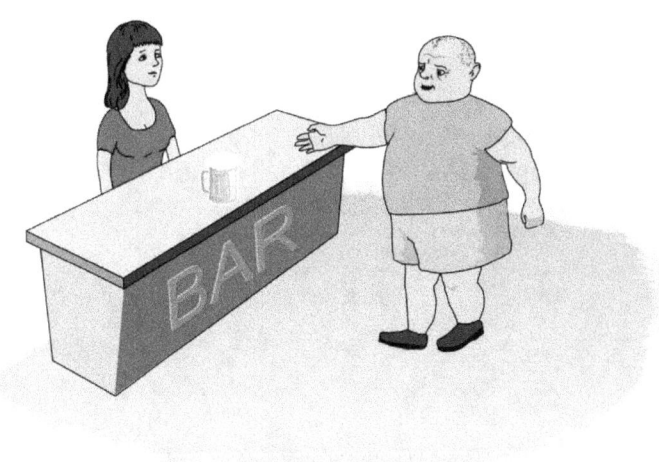

Alcohol is one of the most effective drugs that will compromise your dieting quest for fitness. The reason it is such a diet crasher is that it relaxes your nerves giving a false sense of our reality. It tells our brains everything is going to be all right and makes us feel invincible causing us to make decisions that are sometimes not in our best interest.

Does this mean you have to give up alcohol totally? Absolutely not. You can still drink alcohol occasionally and be effective in fitness. For example, if some that say "there is no way I can give up my two glasses of wine a day" it would still be okay as long as there is a balance. Giving up your two glasses is not necessarily a requirement for you to make. It all depends on the total calorie intake on a daily basis. For example: If you are on a 1,500 a day calorie diet and each glass is approximately 100 calories each then you must simply subtract the number of calories in those two glasses from your total calorie intake. This goes the same for two beers or any other alcoholic drink that you consume. If you consume more than just two drinks consistently this will be detrimental to your fitness goals since subtracting the calories of 4-5 drinks is not only unhealthy however you will find the effects of alcohol will slow you down dramatically. Therefore don't overdo the alcohol consumption and take it easy when you do drink occasionally.

2) Socialization

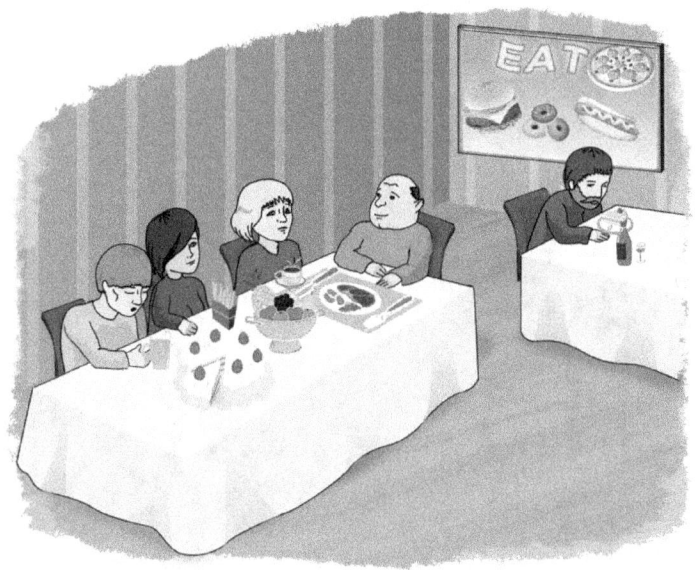

Social environments are sometimes a huge factor in many of our lives. It can be something as simple as a dinner for two or a large event gathering. Eating is generally a part of most social events as part of normal human behavior and is practiced in almost every culture. Unfortunately, there are not always the healthiest choices of food at social events. When you are dining for two you will have more of the advantage of healthy food selections however it will be more difficult at larger events. One way you can battle the cravings when you attend an event that has limited choices is to try to be prepared. Bring an energy bar in your pocket if you must. Eat a small healthy meal before your event. Try to have healthy snack foods available. You will find it much easier to win the battle of cravings if you stay armed.

3) Influence

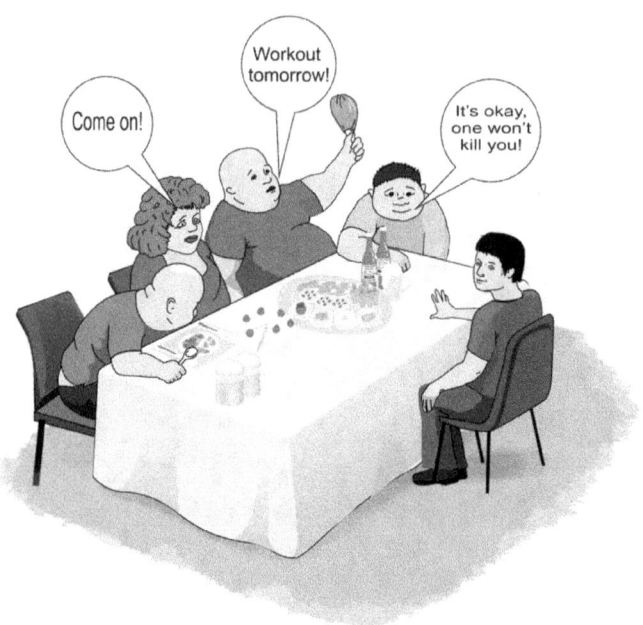

The influence of others will affect your decisions. Remember when you were growing up how you may have been told to watch who you hang around with? You might remember being told in school to not hang around people who do drugs. The reason is due to the natural social outcome called influence and it is extremely powerful. Unless you are going to a social event where everybody is a fitness buff and is serving celery & fat-free yogurt there is no way you will not have the urge to cheat on your diet. If you do not have any trouble and have tremendous discipline then congratulations! However, for most people, they find it difficult if their friends are telling them "come on" "it's okay", "it's a party" "one won't kill you" "just work out tomorrow" etc. The influence of others will affect your decisions if you are not mentally prepared. It is important to be able to tell people: "no thank you but thanks for offering." "I am still full from eating earlier I'll have some later if I get any room." Be genuinely thankful as possible when not letting the influence of others affect us.

4) Celebration

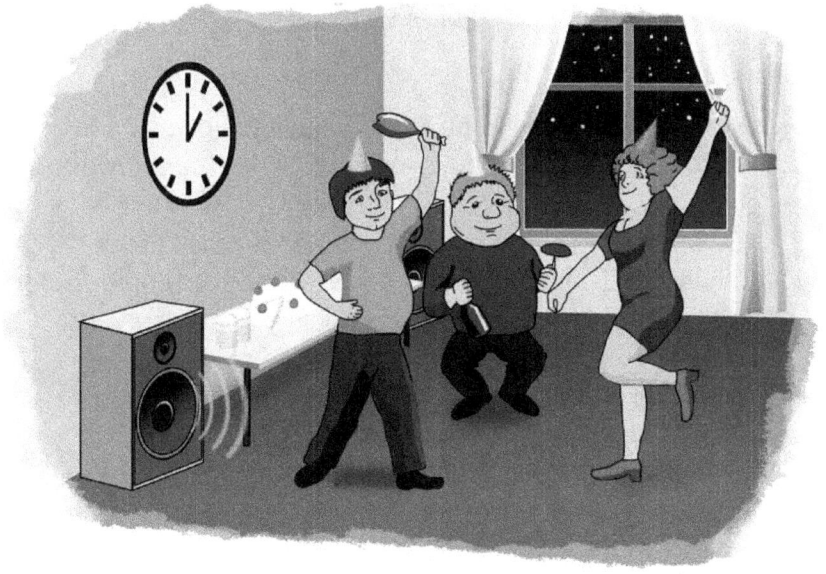

The celebration aspect of the social event is the most difficult to overcome because of course, this is where we generally feel that we owe it to ourselves to do as we please, no matter how unhealthy it can be. As long as you are keeping your celebrations to a limit there is nothing wrong with this. When it comes to celebrating just remember your body belongs to you. It is your property. You cannot necessarily sell or trade it in later for a new one. It belongs to you and your worth is extremely valuable. Try to reverse your mindset so that you have the feeling that caring for your body is deserving of a healthy celebration instead. View your body the same way you would see a new sports car on the showroom floor. Only take it out and open it up every once in awhile to its top speed but never redline it or rag it out. Take care of it and keep it tuned up. Eventually like a fine wine, it will become more valuable as it evolves with age into its antique value. Your body is your vehicle in life getting you where you need to go, so treat your body right. Take care of your property.

View the discipline to be fit as owing it to yourself and your worth. Be the car on the showroom floor. You are worth it.

Determine which events that you will not stick to your fitness goals but splurge as you want and stay on track for the ones that you chose to eat healthy. Visualize your events in advance and this will help you to be more prepared mentally. You may not want to worry about dieting on your birthday or very special occasions but still always remember your worth. Just as you may have one cheat day out of the week as part of your routine you can choose your level of determination of how many celebrations you will splurge.

"Just remember the more wise celebrations you have, the more celebrations you will be able to have. Don't forget to celebrate healthy."

ACTION STEP:

1) Alcohol, Socialization, Influence, and Celebration are the key factors that make up the difference if you stick with your motivation during your social events. Whether if you stay on track using the weekly step system will depend on how many social events you attend and how many you celebrate healthy. An unhealthy celebration will put you back 6 out of the 7-day weekly step system of progress. Therefore if you have two events in one week maintain one as your healthy celebration.

CONCLUSION

Remember with anything moderation is the key. Quite simply put don't party too much, too much of anything will catch up with you. Social events are a part of our life. The company of others stimulates our minds and makes life interesting. Without relationships of others, life can be dull so keeping strong mental health is important to keeping our soul enlightened with joy. Strive to associate with positive people that will support your health goals and you will find staying on track more manageable.

LEAVING THE LAKE PARTY

I'll never forget the time my friends and I took a wrong turn down a country road.

I was 16, just got my driver's license and my big brother who was a young Marine at the time, bought me my first car for $300. It was a white 1979 4-door Impala. I fixed up the interior with supplies I got from Wal-mart. I put in new carpet and had fixed it up enough to be considered cool by the other kids.

One day I was out with my friends and we had just come back from an exotic animal drive-through ranch in the area and took a wrong turn down a country dirt road.

It was almost dark but the sun was still up. We pulled into this dirt road that led up to a farmhouse and saw some people standing outside.

I figured we asked them for directions on how to get back on the main road. As we got closer we realized they were three girls that were our age. We had seen them in school before but never spoke to them.

They came up to our windows to talk and were instantly flirty... "hey, we see you guys at school!"

We got to talking for a bit and my friend said, "hey you want to go out to the lake tomorrow?"

They said yes and we were all excited. That next morning I packed some sandwiches in a cooler and sodas with ice. In those days you could buy a generic brand of sodas from HEB called Plaza and it was only a dollar for 6 cans and they came in all kinds of flavors such as root beer and cream soda.

My friend borrowed his mom's car and we thought we had the hookup and were off to the lake. We had two cars, sandwiches, and Plaza sodas!

We picked up the three girls and rode out to the lake. I remember one of the girls sitting behind me. She kept putting her hand on top of my head feeling my gelled hair telling me how nice it was.

It was a good 30 to 45-minute drive to get there and find the spot we were looking for to swim at.

I remember feeling anxiety as we got out there. Everyone starting stripping getting into their swimwear.

All of a sudden I couldn't do it. I felt paralyzed. I didn't want to strip. My friends already took off their shirts. I wore a nice polo looking shirt trying to look nice for the occasion and it wasn't the kind of shirt you would leave on to swim in without looking ridiculous. I forgot to bring an extra shirt to swim in and I was too shy.

I was so embarrassed and I didn't know what to do. I told my friend, "hey can you all ride back in your car, I'm going to head back."

My friends were shocked. The girls were shocked. I took the cooler out from the trunk with sodas and sandwiches and put them in my friend's car and without explaining the details, I said goodbye. I could hear the girls whispering. "Why is he leaving?"

I was too embarrassed to tell them why and I just wanted to get out of there.

I remember driving back occasionally glancing at myself in my sun visor mirror.

Deep down I hated being overweight.

It was at that time that I realized, this is not who I am.

I didn't want to be fat anymore.

Some day... I told myself. Some day.

Chapter 10

Activating Your Energy Source for Life

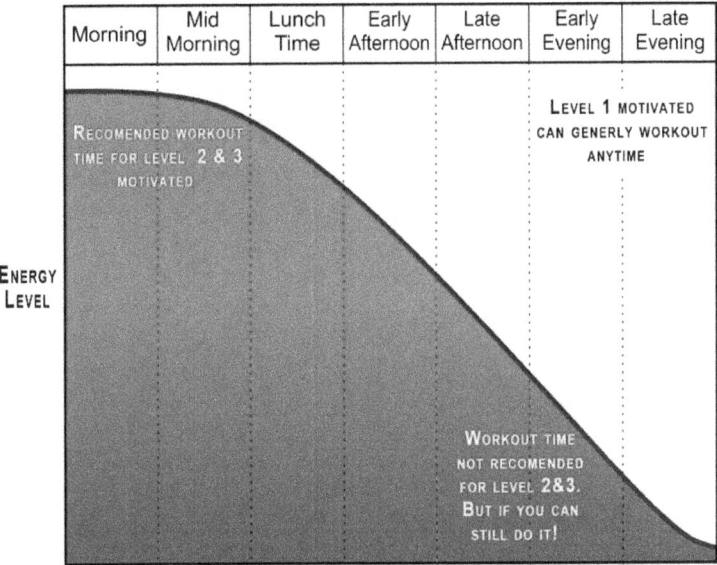

Morning	Mid Morning	Lunch Time	Early Afternoon	Late Afternoon	Early Evening	Late Evening

RECOMENDED WORKOUT TIME FOR LEVEL 2 & 3 MOTIVATED

LEVEL 1 MOTIVATED CAN GENERLY WORKOUT ANYTIME

ENERGY LEVEL

WORKOUT TIME NOT RECOMENDED FOR LEVEL 2&3. BUT IF YOU CAN STILL DO IT!

WORKOUT ENERGY CHART

This shows the importance of why you need to start your exercise ritual early in the morning if possible. The above chart illustrates exercising and shows the energy level times when comparing to motivational levels. After a certain point in the day, your energy begins to decline and if this is your only available work out time then this is the time you have to reach deep within. The energy is there in your heart and your mind. Keep thinking about being sexy on the beach and whatever is important to you. Reach deep and always get it done. The bonus is you are adding years to your life. You can do it.

Time You Work Out

This chapter is going to help you with the physiological approach of motivation that you are going to need to work out. There is an untapped energy source we all have. It's there. It's just up to you if you will reach deep inside and resurrect this energy when it is time to work out, even when you don't feel like it. The following is a breakdown of what we go through when it comes to the process of getting started and also many mental techniques you can use to your advantage.

The Brain Science of Exercise

1) The Warm-Up

This is the time that you must reach within and just get started. It is the opportunity time that separates who will succeed in reaching their goals since it is more difficult to initiate exercise versus if you are already exercising. You may notice when you first start working out that for the first couple of minutes it may seem very difficult. Your body and mind may go into a shock of temporary discomfort. If you are not used to this kind of activity you may be mentally saying to yourself "What am I doing?" "There is no way I can keep this up for 20-30 minutes?!" Remember your joints are cold and your blood is not flowing yet. Remember to give it time because it is simply "temporary discomfort" meaning it won't last the entire time. Think of your body as a working engine. Start even a brand new engine on a cold morning and you will find it still needs warming for optimum performance. It can also not sit for long periods of time without running periodically. A mechanic would recommend an engine to be started up at least every three months. Once it gets warmed up it doesn't run as rough and it can idle. The body can also not just sit and not have activity for long periods for optimum performance. It needs to warm up and get over the period of rough idling. It needs to go through the warm-up phase every time you begin a new workout. Get into your workout and start warming up to idle longer.

Start your engines.

Warm-up!

2) The Point of No Return

Get your RPM's going is a saying also used in the mechanical world. In an engine, this is referred to as revolutions per minute. When relating this to the body it is the same concept however it is your heart rate you need to get going. This is the stage your body feels after getting warmed up. It may be ten minutes for some, for others, it might be 20. It will vary per individual's activity level however, once achieved it will seem much easier to complete the remainder of your work out. The quicker you can reach the point of no return, the faster you can complete the remainder of your workout without the feeling of discomfort. This will allow you to add on an additional 30, 40, or even 50 minutes to your work out. It is called the point of no return because once you start and your body achieves the warmth from the physical activity it reaches a comfort zone. This is the time you will feel unstoppable and it is a great feeling. Different people and different physical levels will vary on how much activity it will take to reach their elevated heart rate. It may just be walking at a fast pace, the elliptical or jogging that does it. Just make sure to reach your point of no return to where it is comfortable and you can get a good workout going. Make sure to get your RPM's revved high and get into your point of no return.

3) The Release!

Get to it! It's like a shot of pure natural high. The body loves it. It thrives on it but the only way it can get there is by getting in the gym and getting the blood to pump through the body. The medical term for it is called endorphins and becoming addicted to them can be the best addiction problem you can ever have. Studies show it will put you in a better mood. No antidepressant pill or supplement can do this more effectively or safely than the body's own natural abilities. It is like God's gift to us that is the body's natural secret. Talk to active fitness individuals and ask them why they are passionate about working out. A good fitness expert will take the time to explain the many reasons why they are always achieving this feeling and how it makes them feel.

4) The Reward

The psychological effect after exercise is complete is the reward stage. Research has proven that people tend to eat better if they have been actively exercising versus if they have not. It is a psychological process of the mind knowing that it is making progress. The reward also plays a factor in the feeling you get as a sense of achievement and accomplishment. It is a combination that works together between the release of endorphins and the relaxation of the body. When you seek out progress to achieve the reward stage of exercise you will also find the reward as an addictive process you will want to add into your regimen and lifestyle for years to come.

Stay active and go through all the stages of the exercise process.

Influence - The Energy From Others

You play golf with better golfers...

Meaning if you are just playing by yourself or with amateurs, you may not take the game as seriously. No one is really holding you accountable and you do not necessarily have the need to play at your best performance.

However, if you were playing with pros, you tend to step up your game. You focus on each swing more and try to make every hole count.

That same influence of energy works the same way in the fitness world. Being in the fitness environment such as fitness centers and surrounding yourself with others who are motivated will help you step up your game to reach your goals faster. If your only opportunity is to work out in your garage then go for it. It is better to work out in some way within your means possible than not to work out at all. Just remember to surround yourself with motivated people whenever possible and view this as an opportunity to play with pros to step up your game.

Feeling Better & Boosting Energy Levels

The boost is the other added incentive of the exercise process. It takes place after you have become conditioned to exercising on a consistent basis. Your body adapts to things it is used to doing. Once it has adapted to doing exercise it will start to crave physical activity. Just as it adapts to consuming large amounts of calories or anything else you condition yourself to do, it conforms to the routine you give it. Once you are conditioned to this level of physical activity you will crave it the day you stop doing it. When you go through this phase it will be rewarding. The energy boost process will make your body feel like a young dog that craves running around outdoors. This is what is referred to as exercising boosting your energy level. No matter what age you begin, exercise is proven to boost any one's energy level at all intervals of life. It is the best-prescribed medicine you can give yourself. You decide if you fill your prescription or not and when you pick it up. It will be the time that you feel energized and better about yourself. It is the time you just want to keep going and enjoy everything life throws your way.

Prescribe yourself with a boosted energy level and fill your prescription often.

Keeping Your Mental Strength Focused During Cardio

While you are training there will be many things going in your mind during cardio. Depending on the level of your physical abilities the required focus will vary of how much mental focus it will take to concentrate to make it through your workouts. For example, when you first start walking at a slow pace, many will find this natural movement fairly easy. However, for some beginners, if you are not used to this activity level for some even slight cardio can be difficult to maintain a good pace. Whatever performance level a person is at you still want to get your activity level to where your heart rate becomes elevated and much of your focus is required to maintain this level. Do not worry, regardless of your activity level ability and gradually work your way to progress into the next pace of walking faster and faster. Your body will build a tolerance of abilities to perform cardio at a more rapid pace in time. However, always make sure to get to the level of activity to where it requires your mind to use a strong mental focus.

How to Motivate Your Mind to Kill Cardio Time

Depending on the level of cardio you are performing as well as your training level you might find it difficult for time to pass until you become accustomed to warming up. If high cardio levels are something you are not used to then your body will need to adapt to it. This will happen with time and consistency of performing exercises. Once you get into the level of an elevated heart rate you will want to keep a pace of mental focus during your exercise session. Think of it as meditation but instead at a rapid heartbeat and air is flowing through your lungs at a faster pace. Initially, when you begin a workout you may be thinking about the amount of time left whether on your stopwatch or watching the timer on a treadmill. Regardless of what time is left you do not want to focus on the fact you have 30-45 minutes left on your workout. You want to focus on the feeling of warmth you are about to feel and how long it is going to take to get there. Once you achieve the feeling of warmth this is the time your body temperature and muscles will, in fact, warm up. For this time to come and pass, time will need to pass. In order for time to pass you need to be somewhat comfortable in your mental focus.

Keep your mind occupied either with thoughts of things that are exciting and comforting to you while keeping enough focus to keep your body going through the motions.

Mind Comfort Level Samples

Songs - Music is one of the most effective ways to make time pass during cardiovascular exercises. The sound of music gets into our nervous system and makes us want to move our bodies. Music can change your mood instantly and change the tone of any environment. Just as the saying what's a party without music the same goes for a good workout. Find your favorites tunes that give you the uplift and put you in a better mood. It's all about connecting your feelings and thoughts so your mind can command your body to get active and moving.

Counting Backwards Slowly - Similar to the way a countdown is on a rocket ship this is something that can be done very slowly. The slow backward count tends to take more time to do however this can make time go by quickly. There's also a psychological factor when counting backward for the progress of what is left to having more clarity of the end. Once you're done start over from the beginning. Try counting back from 100. Before you know it once you have repeated counting backward several times a couple of minutes will have passed quickly.

Thinking about your upcoming weekend - Think about what you will be doing on the weekend or your time off of work. Whether it's playing with the kids or doing something exciting, getting caught up in the thoughts of your plans takes your mind off of discomfort while getting your body warm.

Watching T.V. - Many gyms nowadays offer t.v.'s built right into the cardio equipment. Just make sure to find something that is entertaining and you enjoy watching to let the time pass. Before you know it you may find yourself laughing and feeling in a good mood making your cardio time feel natural.

Concentrate on Your Stride - The stride concentration is something to do easily while walking, jogging, or running. When you have a clear focus of the sole movements of your legs it is similar to the hypnosis process. You will have the ability to go through the motions and focus more on keeping your pace.

Pretending Your Body Is a Machine - Think of your body as a vehicle and you are driving the transportation from the brain.

Concentrate On Your muscles - Focus on the muscles in your legs. Visualize the leg muscles are pistons in an engine ignited with the food you ate earlier as fuel.

All these are psychological samples to help assist you to kill time and maintain your mental focus when doing cardio. Find what works for you. Before you know it time will pass and you will breeze through your workout sessions with ease and gain endurance.

Resistance training or weight lifting is an example of an

anaerobic exercise meaning without oxygen. Aerobic is with oxygen and is more rhythmic. Both anaerobic and aerobic will take mental focus and you just have to find what works for you to get your blood pumping.

Focus: Brain/Nerves
Body: Muscles/Joints
Conditioning: Lungs/Heart

Remember having the visuals of all of these components working together assist your mental strength and your nervous system to make the difference. Arnold Schwarzenegger was known for saying things like, "When I am curling my mind is inside my bicep." He would visually imagine himself going inside his muscle, fully focusing on the repetitions.

This is why these physiological visuals are also so important for cardio as well. Practice and exercise them and your mind will begin to push your body.

ACTION STEPS:

1) Warming Up - Visualize and complete the warm-up before you start exercising hard. If you rev an engine high in the cold morning you risk damaging the future performance of the engine. Take care of your body and prevent injury.

2) Use Psychological Visuals - You will perform better when you surround yourself with positive people.

3) Prescribe Yourself an Energy Boost - How much exercise you do will boost your energy level and you will feel better. This will happen when you are not working out and your body starts to crave physical activity. Feeling energized is just another added incentive.

4) Use Psychological Visuals - When you start your exercise sessions use visuals to keep your mental focus high to achieve longer workout sessions. Use this mental focus to get warmed up and kill time. Use different techniques to find a balanced ability to focus into contentment in conjunction with having a rapid heart rate. This is key to being able to accomplish the maximum workouts your body is capable of performing for long periods of time.

CONCLUSION

Now that you have a crystal clear understanding of the exercise process you will know what is taking place physically and mentally. When we have a better understanding of how things work we can leverage the knowledge to make improvements. Utilize this knowledge to achieve maximum workouts, again and again, and it will improve how you feel and look for the rest of your life.

Chapter 11

Weight Loss After Pregnancy

Several women were interviewed while writing to complete this chapter. If you are pregnant, have just given birth, or a mom at any size. The information here is of great value and will help your weight loss journey regardless of where you are. Men. DO NOT skip this chapter because in a partner relationship it is essential to work together. If you are a man that is single but one day plans to be married and have children then you will want to read forward.

Giving birth to a child is the most beautiful gift women have as humans. Women have been blessed with this gift of giving life and opportunity to give back. We should all embrace this special gift of life as a time to give back. It is also an opportunity for us to remember that along with giving life comes the responsibility to protect it. One of the important elements is to demonstrate to our young how to live the most fulfilled life as possible. This begins with health.

This chapter is intended to give you encouragement, perspective on your mindset and ideas on how to achieve weight loss during, and after pregnancy, however, it is important to note that not everyone loses weight the same way or in the same amount of time. That being said, I want to stress that YOU ARE BEAUTIFUL no matter what the scale says because you were made in the image of God. Weight loss is not so much about the looks as it is about the health reasons. God blessed you with a child so it is up to

you to keep your longevity of health so that you may enjoy your children and possible grandchildren or even great-grandchildren. Stay focused and know that you are beautiful, and you are worthy of a healthy life.

Below are three reasons why it is important for you to strive to be a fit mom and live a healthy lifestyle after pregnancy.

Reason 1)

It Is Wise to Lead By Example

When discussing the acts of nature in chapter two here is an example in reference to how we are creatures of nature. Think back to the examples of our lions once again in chapter two and think about the mother lions raising her cubs. The mother lion must be able to show her young how to hunt for food. She must be fast and demonstrate strength, agility, and stamina. If she is unable to complete this act of nature then her cubs will never learn the fundamental survival techniques they need and the mother will risk how her cubs will succeed in the world. This natural act of nature relates to humans, as we must demonstrate in our lives how to help our young to succeed. We must be smart, wise, and have the ability to perform. Our performance in the world reflects how we take care of ourselves. We are like a nurturing life filter that begins at the top from our parenting. When we are healthier we feel better and we when feel better the possibilities are an endless amount of opportunities of fulfillment.

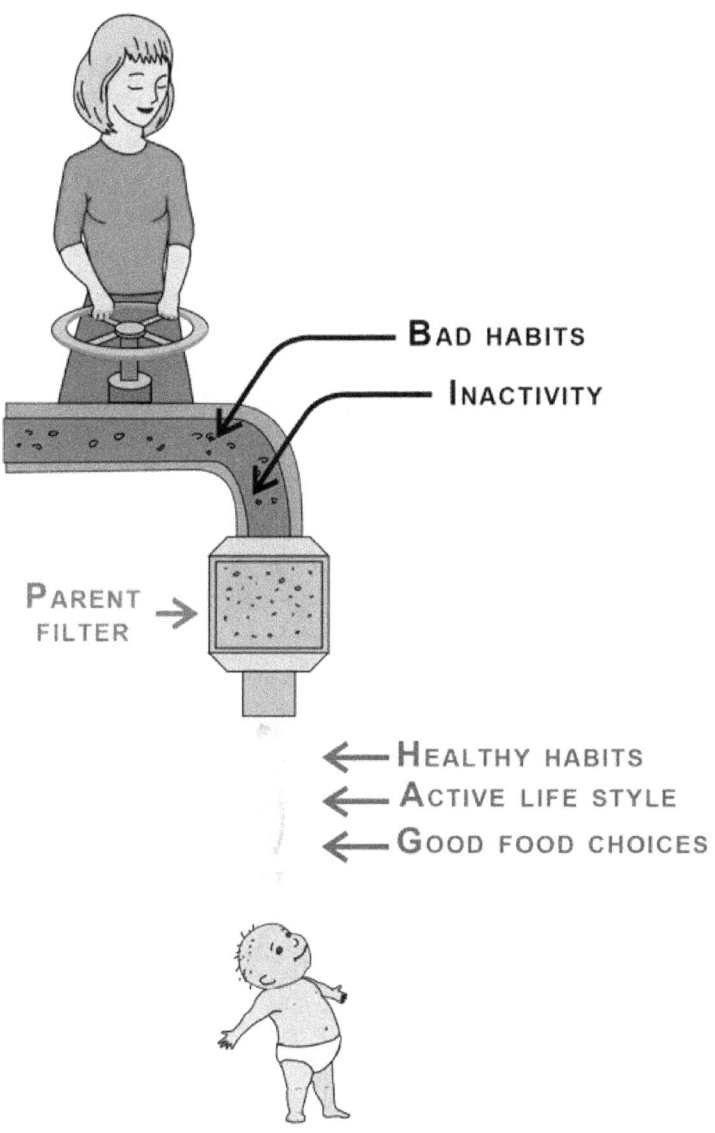

Remember why fitness is an important fundamental trait of life that is essential to your young. Set the best example you can give and demonstrate to them to live the most fulfilling life they can live for themselves.

Remember how judgmental society is and how competitive the world will be for our children. Job interviews, selections in opportunities and competitions for achievements will always revolve around their health and ability to perform. By leading by example to be fit you are demonstrating the importance to them just as the mother lion demonstrates to her cubs.

A wise decision is to lead by example.

Reason 2)

It Is Healthier

It is a wise decision to be healthier after pregnancy and here is why. You should not just strive to eventually be a healthy grandma but a healthy great-grandma!

This is the mindset we need to have as parents. Life spans are now increasing and it's time to enjoy the world's progressions of beauty and all its technological advances that allow us to live longer. When you look into your children's eyes it should inspire you to want to be healthy for them many years to come. Becoming healthier after pregnancy is a wise decision. Remember you are beautiful and tenacious, strong enough to have a child. You are strong enough to lose the weight you want, when you want.

Keep referring to this motivational book when needed to gain the extra motivational knowledge you need. You can do it.

Reason 3)

The Time Is Now

Time is imperative when trying to bounce back after pregnancy. Many view this as a window of opportunity. The initial phase after you have your baby is one of the most effective phases your body will go through with its weight loss capabilities at its prime. Your body is going through dramatic changes to bounce back to its normal state returning to natural comfort. Think of the momentum of your body's natural hormone cycle like a huge tidal wave coming through. If you are able to get on and ride this wave you will have a very strong chance of having effective results in achieving the body you previously had before. Even if you did not have the body you desired initially before pregnancy this is the perfect opportunity to take advantage of this time. If time has passed and you are already past this phase then remember, it is never too late. It only gets harder as more time passes and the longer your body carries the extra weight it will not get any easier therefore "the time is now".

Although your body may not have its same shape as before never give up the battle and never surrender to settling for what you are not happy with. You deserve to be a prominent proud mother reflecting the beauty not only on the inside but also on the outside. Regardless of how long it has been since you have had your pre-pregnancy body the time to act is now. It will all start how you feel on the inside so that your actions of respect for yourself will act upon as if you are in charge of your destiny to achieve the physical happiness you desire. You make that decision along with the choices you make.

Take the approach of not "how" or "if" but instead "<u>when</u>" and "<u>how much</u>" weight will I lose. Start using the power of your mind to make you start taking action and realize the time is now.

Phases of Thoughts - What is going through your mind during pregnancy.

The First Realization

Now that you have a better understanding of the reasons to lose weight after pregnancy it's time to understand some of the phases of thoughts you may go through.

If you are in shape and just found out you're pregnant then it is obvious that you know that you will be gaining weight soon. Soon you will find these thoughts shifting from selfishness, of "what is going to happen to my body?" soon start to shift to naturally focus on your baby and motherhood. Your natural instincts kick in and somewhere along the line many women forget what life was like before pregnancy and view their pre-pregnancy bodies as something in the past.

- It is during this motherly thinking period of beginning to shift and plan for the future that it is easy for many to forget they need to be thinking of the importance to stay healthy. This period of motivation to eat nutritional foods must stay strong and the mental strength to lose weight after the pregnancy must remain an active thought while going through this transformation.

During your pregnancy, you should eat whenever you are hungry and listen to your body when it tells you that you're hungry. Listen to your body, not your mind or what people are telling you how much you should eat. In other words, you should eat slightly more than you should because your body is naturally craving the extra nutrients and food resourcefulness.

Your cravings are sometimes going to be out of control than they normally would. Still be smart and if you must indulge, try to indulge healthy when possible. This is the beginning of giving your child the healthy nutrients it needs.

Overall do not stress about gaining weight while pregnant and embrace it. Just know deep down that when the time comes to focus on losing weight after you have your baby that will be the right time. As long as you maintain these thoughts in your peripheral focus of the near future then your subconscious thoughts will train your mind to be a weight-losing machine when that time comes.

Stages - The Different Types of Health Conscious Moms

The Novice Fitness Mother: This mother does not practice the normal increase in eating cycles you go through as a mother and instead excessively indulges. This mom cares deeply however, she might have fallen victim to the myth of eating for two during pregnancy. Being fit may not have been a priority in her life. During your pregnancy, you should eat whenever you are hungry and when your body tells you to. In other words, you should eat slightly more than you should because your body is naturally craving extra food. Satisfy your natural cravings and ensure your cravings are fulfilled so that you can ensure you have enough nutrients for your baby. However, it is important not to fall into the habit that you must eat excessively whenever you want and whatever you want.

Remember you will still need to bounce back after your pregnancy is over. This mother generally wants and desires to lose weight after pregnancy but simply may be dealing with the many tasks of life and being a mom for other children as well. Change is possible and if you find yourself in this category it is okay because the fact that you have made the decision to read this book at this very moment already shows you have what it takes to improve so give yourself a pat on the back. Take a deep breath and realize you have what it takes to get your pre-pregnancy body back.

The Intermediate Fitness Mother: This mother is generally a naturally fit mother before her pregnancy and loses her shape during pregnancy. About 50% of the time she is able to bounce back depending on her age, life's environment and sphere of influence, however, regardless she generally always maintains the desire to get back to where she was before pregnancy at all times. The intermediate fitness mother is usually always trying.

The Advance Fitness Mother: This mom will generally bounce back quickly and jumps back into the routine habits of fitness as if she fell off a horse. She realizes her health habits are important to her and her thought process is to distinctly reach her goals as soon as she has the ability. She might have learned this valuable lifestyle trait early on from her own mother or at some point she decided that it would be her priority. She tries to view herself as a healthy mom is a good mom and can generally be found staying active regardless.

Some moms not only view fitness for them just after pregnancy as important but they also visualize themselves with their babies growing older and being a fit mom. Visualizing their kids getting older, attending their activities and being proud of them as a fit mother are all healthy visuals. All moms generally want this and it is healthy to also visualize your future desires.

Your children deserve to have you as the fittest, healthiest mom possible. Become the fittest mom you can be and begin demonstrating this choice of life so that your children will see this from a very early stage of childhood. They will mirror neuron and mimic you.

After all, they are you.

Below are thoughts from moms from all fitness levels during pregnancy and after, that are striving to be fit:

What a woman is thinking during the different trimesters and what exactly is going through her mind about trying to maintain her health after pregnancy?

Q: What is a woman going through? **A: *During each trimester? or after having a baby? I can only remember what it felt like after having a baby. And what it felt like being pregnant. I cannot remember each trimester. All I can remember is that I was always tired, hungry and anxious about the unknown, worried***

all the time if things were going right and preparing things for when the baby arrived. I read up on what to do how to prepare and I nested all the time. Some days you feel happy and some days you just wanted the baby out! I think those were from all the changing hormones. I found myself overwhelmed at times reading all the self-help and information out there. It wasn't until my second child that I felt more relaxed about having a baby.

During my second pregnancy, I did better on weight gain and I did not gain as much weight because I was more relaxed. I knew what was coming and I knew what was going to happen. I was an emotional eater. Emotional eaters usually eat more when they are nervous, anxious, and sad. After baby #1 I was so focused on the baby that I did not even care about myself. I lost some weight only because I did not have time to eat taking care of the baby. That is when I found myself low on milk production and I realized that I had to eat right to produce milk. For me getting back to a healthy weight was way on the back burner for a while. I think I started thinking of myself after the first year. And that was a lot of yo-yo dieting. After the second child again the focus was on the child not me and there were a lot of medical concerns with the second child. I did not start thinking about my health and then 4 months after my second child my health failed me and I was in the hospital fighting for my life. And I made it, it was then I vowed to stay healthy for my children. And make sure they would grow up healthy as well as eating the right foods. I vowed to feed my children with only healthy foods and cook healthy.

And till this day I still am trying to make healthy choices. I may not be the size I want to be but I am always trying to make healthy choices like taking a walk before sitting down to watch TV, cooking a healthy meal instead of going out to eat fast food. Buying fruits and vegetables, cooking and feeding healthier choices to my children every day starting at a young age. My battle of getting to a healthier weight is a constant struggle and my children see that, and I am hoping that they learn a lesson from my struggles. I can say they are healthy and do make healthy choices, I have been lucky.

Q: How do you feel? **A:** *when pregnant? BIG, Hungry, Tired! NOT SEXY!*

Q: How does a woman keep her motivation when she is stuck with the extra weight after pregnancy and <u>what can she do to keep a positive state of mind during this time</u>? **A:** *Support system from your spouse and your friends, finding a buddy to walk with you or talk to about your plan. Talking with your spouse about your plans and having your spouse help you with your goals and plans is very helpful and important. Making small attainable goals, goals that can be met easily, then move on to the next one eventually leading to your big main goal. For example, my goal might be to walk two miles every day for a month and then next month walk 3 miles. Your goals don't always have to be weight loss it could be a fitness level or my goal might be to fit into a certain favorite dress by Christmas. Last finding motivation from your children is always a sure thing, they always seem to motivate you especially if they are old enough, you can share your goals with* *them and get them involved. For example, you might ask your older children can you remind me to take my walks every day and will you go with me if I don't have someone to go with? Your children will either be happy to go or will not let you forget. You are doing three things you are teaching them to be compassionate, helpful, and you are teaching them to think of others besides themselves. Oh, and you are also teaching them the importance of staying healthy.*

Thoughts from a fitness mom and things she thinks of to keep her fitness motivation:

Pregnancy is not only an emotional time for the new expectant mother but for the father to be as well. It is just the cold, hard truth that with the beauty of pregnancy comes the maternity jeans, oversized tops, and spandex pants that for some reason seem to be a permanent fixture in a new mother's wardrobe long after the new little addition has made its debut.

The miracle of carrying a child is physically as well as emotionally trying for a new mom. Not only is there the emotional roller coaster that has to be ridden non-stop for nine months, but there is also the extra 30 pounds that are gained. It would be a nice, perfect world if every woman felt that she was "glowing" during her pregnancy, but for most women, while that may actually be the case, they do not feel that way. With the heartburn, backaches, excruciating hot weather, and aching feet, the last thing that a woman feels is beautiful. While the miracle of bearing a child and becoming a mother is life-changing, the weight gain is not a picnic for any woman.

I have heard countless women say that they were "fat" during their pregnancy, when in fact they were gaining the weight that was intended. A strong support system during pregnancy is key.

For women, it is so easy to give in to those cravings while pregnant with the stigma "I am eating for two" justifying that extra piece of cake or pint of cherry garcia in the middle of the night. But men this is where a strong support system is your bread and butter. With all of the emotions troubling a pregnant woman, a stable motivated father-to-be is a key ingredient to staying on the motivational track during pregnancy. A woman should gain anywhere from 25 to 35 pounds during her pregnancy. Anything above that is in excess. That is weight that no woman wants to gain. The extra 10 pounds on top of the "baby weight" is what keeps new moms in the maternity jeans. By staying motivated while pregnant and still leading a healthy lifestyle including smart food options and safe exercise, that extra weight can be avoided. Taking steps to prevent that dreaded "I never lost the baby weight" line after 12 months post-pregnancy, is a sure-fire way to keep a life of motivation rolling during the adventure of pregnancy. With a new baby, weight is most likely to be that last thing on any new mom's mind. But once a routine gets in place and mom starts to break out those old "skinny" jeans, reality can sink in. When those go-to jeans are no longer able to button post-pregnancy, many women react in different ways.

A new baby for some is all the motivation in the world

to lose that extra bit of weight. Being in shape and healthy for your kids is a very positive way to get back in the swing of things and back into those skinny jeans. However, for some women, the reality of gaining so much weight can really take its toll. Postpartum depression is a serious condition in which a new mom may often feel sad or depressed which hinders the ability to move forward. Fathers, your role as a supportive spouse and positive influence is crucial at a time like this. New moms are just as new to the game as you are and can become overwhelmed just as easy. Having a good team together can make the transition easier for both of you. There is always the old age excuse that can result to NEVER losing the baby weight. It is sad to say, but when there is a toddler running around, that is no longer baby weight. This is where pregnancy is no longer the culprit in the prevention of reaching your fitness goals. Coming out of the denial that the extra weight you are carrying is not, in fact, baby weight is the key to beginning a new life. Admitting to yourself is the first step to success and what could be more motivating than getting back into your skinny jeans. That pre-pregnancy bod is not out of reach with the right steps, support, and motivation to be the most positive influence you can be for yourself as well as your new little addition.

Thoughts from a Veteran Mom:

With both my girls I did nothing but think about their needs and did not have the self-worth of taking care of myself. I accepted that my role was solely taken care of them, my husband, the house, etc... Society, family, friends, played into the guilt I felt if I took time out for myself. Now that I am older and wiser, I realize that my health is just as important and that I am doing my children an injustice if I don't take care of me so that I can take care of them.

While I was pregnant I did, however, make sure to eat the right things because I wanted a healthy child, but using the excuse that I am "eating for two" was not the right choice and it was a myth. I know that now. Losing the baby weight after birth for me was not a priority; my focus was mainly bringing up healthy children. I now know that if I want healthy children I have to be a role model and reflect to them a healthy lifestyle. How can I expect them to make the right food choices if I am not eating the right foods myself?

ACTION STEPS:

1) **Understand Your REASONS OF WHY -** Having a crystal clear vision of the reasons of your motivation as a mom helps you to have complete certainty. When you become a parent it makes you into a protector of your children to where nothing will stop your assurance and drive to provide prosperity into their lives. Realize that for this to be at its fullest you deserve to live healthy beside them.

2) **Become The Role Model -** for your children so that they can be guided down a healthy path and ensure the parent filter stays on for their future.

3) **Understand the different levels of fitness moms** - You now have information to give you perspective

on the different levels of fitness moms as well as have heard their different feedback approaches to fitness. Notice the tough love approach from the thoughts of a fitness mom. Write down all your excuses as well as all the reasons you should strive to be fit. Review them both and take the time to reflect. Make the decision. You got this mom.

CONCLUSION: Moms come in all shapes in the form of love. When it comes to fitness, it is a decision and there is no room for excuses. You are a beautiful loving mother that gave life and has what it takes. That love is strength and you can accomplish anything you want.

FOR MEN: SUPPORT AND LOVE MOMS STRIVING TO BE FIT. YOUR PATIENCE, LOVE, AND SUPPORT MAKE ALL THE DIFFERENCE.

Chapter 12

Using Supplements to Boost Your Mental Motivation

Safe supplements can be good when used correctly and wisely. One of the most effective ways to satisfy your cravings can be by utilizing supplements. Protein shakes, energy bars, and even some dietary supplements can help you. Use these supplements to boost your motivation. Don't rely on them.

Supplements come in different forms such as: physical, consumables and mental. You may be a strong-willed and determined person however this book is an example of motivational content that will help supplement even a very highly motivated person's mentality. Sometimes we just need a little boost to help us and that's what supplements do. They help us with our diet, recovering and even mental motivation. When it comes to consumable supplements such as diet remedies and food supplements, you have to do your homework to make sure that what you are using is proven, effective and most of all safe. The good thing with today's technology is even if you don't have people at your side to ask their input you can become an expert on things you want to know by doing your online homework. When it comes to consumable supplements they can help you but it is ALWAYS worth the time to do your detailed research on them.

Diet Pills

There is no magic pill. There are many weight loss

products on the market to include thermogenics which are basically pills that are also referred to as fat burners. Make sure you read outside the labels about the products you are thinking about taking. Fat burners are basically thermogenics that generally have large doses of caffeine in them which in turn will generally give you an energy boost. This energy boost will usually result in you being less hungry and also feeling energized to work out.

Keep in mind you are putting a tremendous amount of stress on your nervous system and any fat burner pill should be taken with caution and never over the recommended dosage.

In the long run, just simply remember. Without proper nutrition and exercise, it makes no sense to take any diet pills. Supplements should be used just as that. As supplements, not solutions. Be smart, strategic, and methodical when taking supplements. Don't be the victim resulting in a case study of a dangerous side effect. You can lose weight with fat burner pills but be cautious. If you find you must try these supplements try to taper off as soon as possible and only use them to give you a boost to get started but once you get on track to your weight loss, you got this! Reach deep inside to harness your natural fat-burning abilities and reap the reward of longevity instead. It would be counterproductive to your fitness goals to take the supplements long term only to do damage to your overall health.

Just remember there is no magic pill that is going to supplement a proper diet and exercise, however, when you combine supplements with your fitness regiment they can assist you to create faster results. When you see faster results you gain more psychological motivation.

But once you get on track to weight loss always remember longevity is more important. The body is not meant to take that kind of stress on your nervous system consistently. Try not to take pills and get off them soon if you do.

Supplement Technique for Recovery - Massage

Massage is not necessarily a physical supplement you take however it is a supplemental way to recover your muscles from intense workouts and exercise. Just as muscle-relaxing drugs can be used to relax sore muscles a therapeutic massage can do a more effective job. Many people underestimate the power of massage and the physical benefits it brings. They do not realize how effective it can be with its advantages to speed the recovery time up that your body needs to recuperate for longer and harder exercise. Even if you cannot afford a professional massage therapist there are many resources & videos available online to assist someone that can help you with this.

This is when it's great to have a partner so you can help each other. Trade efforts. You scratch my back and I scratch yours is a great concept when you both have fitness goals that you can accomplish together and strengthen your relationship.

The Benefits of Massage

- **Relax** and soften tired, injured, exhausted muscles
- **Improve** the condition of the body's largest organ—the skin.

- **Alleviate Pain** - Improve range of motion and alleviate low-back pain
- **Increase** and allow more joint flexibility.
- **For Expectant Mothers** - Assist with shorter labor, contributes to make easier and shortens maternity hospital stays.
- **Ease** medication dependence.
- **Mental Health** - Lessen anxiety, depression and assist with your overall mood
- **Releases** endorphins and amino acids that work as the body's natural painkiller
- **Stretches** weak, tight, muscles that may be atrophied from nerve damage
- **Relieve migraine** pain
- **Helps Cramping** to relieve and reduces spasms
- **Helps Medically** - Can help with reducing post-surgery adhesions and excessive swelling
- **Circulation** - Helps to increase circulation by pumping oxygen and nutrients into tissues and vital organs.
- **Immune System** - Helps enhance overall immunity by stimulating lymph flow, which is the body's natural defense system.
- **Helps Regenerate** - to promote tissue regeneration, reducing scar tissue and stretch marks.
- **Feels Great** - Plus it feels so good that even deep tissue work can be like an acquired good pain to go through. Endure this pain and your body will thank you after.

Running or jogging, for example, will cause the muscles to tense up and create tension in the back and shoulders. By resting and allowing a day or two for the body to recuperate you allow the body to take on the activity again. By having a therapeutic massage done you speed up this process immensely. When you are able to utilize the advantages of massage as a supplemental recovery technique you can perform better at your weight loss goals. Massage can be your supplement to feeling better and is a technique many bodybuilders and athletes use to train their bodies. Many people underestimate the benefits of massage and its ability to lead them to optimized performance in exercise.

When the body is feeling better it will perform better. When it performs better it will improve more. This momentum continues on and before you know it you are craving the ability to get out and expend your energy. No matter what age or level of fitness. We all have the ability to feel better.

Food Supplements

These are generally fantastic supplements that you can use to feel full and help your motivation. There are many great protein shakes, bars and health supplements on the market that are starting to taste great when you mix with different fruits and experiment with flavors.

It is is very valuable when you become used to drinking a late-night shake to curb hunger pains. When you can do this and conquer the late-night hunger bug you have made a huge achievement. You have now gained a valuable skill in your arsenal to help with the weight loss war.

So the next time it's late and you already ate a lean dinner that was light but not filling. If you are still craving something at night, drink a protein shake. Combined with routine exercise and resistance training, just remember, the voices will soon be heard. "Wow, you are looking great!" "Have you been losing weight!" will make it all worth it.

Cookie Diet

www.cookiediet.com and https://ozhealthpharma.com.au/product-category/cookie-diet/ is a place where you can order diet cookies. They can be ordered by an individual box or in a variety pack and are generally less expensive when compared to the money you spend on food. These cookies do not taste like a regular loaded cookie with sugars and calories however depending on your flavor preference you may find something that is appealing. Probably the biggest benefit to these cookies is the fact that with water they keep you feeling full. Follow the instructions and be sure to take multivitamins. These cookies can be another resource to your arsenal to combat hunger.

Drugs

Steroids or illegal enhancement supplements

They make no sense. They do work. You can take them with limited side effects under a doctor's supervision however why risk this? Unless you are a professional bodybuilder and depend on your physique to make a living and depend on placing number one in the national fitness pageant to depend on your income it just does not make any sense to take away from your longevity just to get the boost for your everyday normal life.

Imagine taking some nitro octane booster and putting it into a race car. This makes sense. It will help the car win the race but of course, the car will eventually be ragged out and must be replaced. The race car drivers will simply jump in another vehicle for their next race. Remember your body is the sports car on the showroom floor. You are the driver. Don't put this stuff in your body. Maybe if you are trying to place number one in a bodybuilding competition for a living but it just does not make any sense.

Be the fit elderly person with the attractive physique on the cruise ship traveling the world enjoying your activities with your grandchildren. Don't be the ragged out race car.

Your body belongs on the showroom floor.

ACTION STEPS:

Use supplements to assist you but not as the magic pill. They will help you speed up progress however it needs to only be a mental boost in your efforts.

CONCLUSION

Be smart. Be wise. You got this.

SHIRTS OR SKINS?

At soccer practice we did small scrimmage games. They were broken down into small groups of 5-7 players on each team and occupied the sections of our large practice field.

We would play each other in groups for about 15 minutes

and then the whistle would blow and we would alternate playing the next group. It was fun practice.

Across from the field was a large parking lot that at times was sectioned off. Occasionally when it was sectioned off some of the high school marching band would practice their routine.

There was a girl that I had a crush on. She played the flute and had the most beautiful smile. She had the kind of personality where she was always laughing and smiling and took a genuine interest when talking to others. Somehow I was able to pull off getting her phone number and would call her at home after school.

I remember always watching to see if I could see her at band practice and see if I could see her looking checking out soccer class.

I remember calling her up one day after school and she said, "hey, I saw you playing at soccer." It made me have a big cheesy smile, I was so proud to be considered athletic. She said, "I have to go, my mom is calling me."

Me, "alright maybe I'll see you at school tomorrow."

I wasn't the best looking kid but I had a charming personality and loved talking to girls on the phone.

The next day I was ready for soccer class and was excited to play. I thought I would play my best so I could impress my girl crush. However, this day did not go as planned though because when we were divided up in groups we had to have shirts and skins.

This means that one group takes off their shirts to identify themselves as a team and the other group leaves their shirts on.

Usually, I would just get lucky and get shirts but if I did get skins, I didn't do as good playing and I dealt with it.

The problem was I just found out that my girl crush could see me from their band practice. All I was thinking was, what if I get skins? I remember coach calling out as he divided the groups and started pointing to each group... Shirts!...Skins!...Shirts!...Skins!

I remember thinking, please let me be shirts, please, please...

And before you know it as coach alternated, the group next to me got shirts... And as he called on my group, I closed my eyes and I could hear.. Skins! :-/

I remember I was so shy, ashamed and embarrassed and all I could think about is what if she looks over at me. I'm going to be running around the field and my fat is going to be jiggling.

I took off my shirt and dealt with it.

I didn't play well. As I would run to kick the ball I subconsciously kept my arms close to my body and didn't feel confident.

All I could think about is what if she is watching me? I tried to play my best but I let my mind get distracted about how I looked without a shirt and it showed in my performance.

I remember getting home and I was too embarrassed to call her. All I could think about is what if she saw me and laughed? I kept thinking negative thoughts and I didn't want to call her.

Next thing... my phone rang. I was hesitant to answer and waited before I picked up.

I slowly picked up the phone... "Hello".. It was her. She said, "Hey, I didn't see you at soccer class, how was your day?"

I was extremely relieved and felt lucky she didn't see me. We talked about other things kids talk about and I avoided about soccer.

The next time we were at practice, my group got shirts. I played hard. I ran. I kicked the ball hard. I played my best.

As I reflect back I realize how silly it was to not play my best because of a shirt.

The shirt was a supplement. Supplements are great. Vitamins, energy boosters, etc.

Most of the time they are physiological. I had it deep inside me to play hard even without a shirt. The shirt gave me confidence.

Most people have it deep within them and carry their own psychological barriers that prevent them from performing.

The next time you are exercising or performing remember, whether if you have a supplement or not, do your best. Use them as a confidence builder when needed but realize you have it deep inside you to perform your best with or without supplements.

Don't get distracted and worry about what people are thinking about you when working out in the gym. Don't worry about what others think about you when trying to perform.

Because deep down, with supplements or not, you have it inside you, to be the best that you can be.

Chapter 13

The Cold Hard Truth

Judgmental Society

Are you concerned about what others think and how they see you? See these samples and scenarios of a judgmental society so that you can learn how to gain the mental strength to overcome them.

Remember,

"You are a vibration of your own frequency that you decide to project to the world."

Admitting The Truth About Society

We live in a judgmental society. There is just no easy way to put it and we must admit the truth about this if we chose to have an accurate awareness of our reality. Many people that are not necessarily judgmental people can easily catch themselves judging others subconsciously without even thinking about it. We're human; it's sometimes just natural. The fact is we all have the same opportunity to live healthy. Just as the people that strive for success and wealth will reap the rewards and benefits of that freedom lifestyle it is the same scenario for those who strive to live fit. Those that make the decision to do this will reap the benefit. You have already taken a huge step towards your health to read this book, therefore, reap the benefits and join the positive side of society's judgments.

You deserve to live longer, feel more energized and look your best. And if the reality is that our society is judgmental then you deserve to live in the benefit of judgment in a positive perception because judgment goes both ways. Negative and positive judgment.

Just as the same way people tend to view overweight people in a negative sense many of those same people will view beautifully fit people in a positive light as attractive. Nothing can be sexier when you see a beautiful person with an amazing glowing personality just owning who they are.

You deserve to feel better.

Jobs

It is shameful to admit however as many people that do not want to admit it the weight factor makes a difference in how we sometimes perform in society. In the job world for instance, unfortunately, it can play a key role. Studies have shown that when you take a group of overweight individuals and compare them to a group of other individuals with similar qualifications that are not overweight, the not overweight group statistically will be hired more.

The majority of employers tend to view how one takes care of their body as how they might perform if given work task. Since losing and maintaining a healthy weight requires discipline many employers will assume that overweight people will lack the same discipline in the workplace. This, of course, is an inaccurate assumption and is completely false however the data reflects a different outlook that should not be ignored in the real world. Additionally, this should be another motivation factor why you should want to reach your goals of the body you envision for yourself.

The other principle that influences these stats is the physical attraction appearance which many times is a factor in the customer service industry or any positions dealing with people. Many employers have good intentions however; subconsciously make decisions without even realizing they are letting appearance determine their hiring decisions. Much of this is already known to most of us however the reality is usually never faced head-on. For example, how many parents teach their children growing up that they need to stay fit so they can ensure they do well in society. This type of thinking is frowned upon for many since the inner beauty quality is supposed to be a priority.

If we are naive to the reality of our society then we will be naive to the results we are getting back in life. You deserve the best opportunities.

Embrace & Change

What is being successful and happy? Should you look in the other direction and not acknowledge the facts of life or should you make the decision to embrace the truth? By taking the step to embrace you are adapting to what is necessary in today's world.

Let's say you are in the stone age of caverns and the times of daily hunting of food. Would being obese allow you to provide the best resources for your loved ones?

Maintaining fitness is imperative in today's world just as it was back then. It has just evolved into a more psychological factor than a physiological one. Take a moment to think about what this means and why it is so important in our modern world.

Relationships- Supply and Demand

The Scale Factor

It is sad to look at things in this way or to even read them on paper however; it goes back to exactly what the name of what chapter 13 is about. You might recall hearing how younger individuals will sometimes refer to others of the opposite sex by relating their levels of attractiveness to a scale. Although juvenile and immature the reality is this is how our society's younger minds sometimes think as they are developing. They are only expressing themselves in the way they know how until they get older and are taught to contain this expressiveness. It is this containment that is, in fact, the mature decision, however, the reality of the internal feelings of how we judge others are still there and it's simply never discussed.

For example, if someone is extremely attractive they are considered a 10 on a scale of 1 to 10 with 10 being the highest level of attractiveness and 1 being the least. If they are unattractive they are considered a 1. Sadly but true this type of thinking starts at a very young age. Many parents do a great job of guiding their children to accept people for who they are as people however it is a battle every day with many younger minds. Once again the pre-programming factor is emphasized with model magazines, cover girl commercials and television shows/movies that mold our young minds early in life. These pre-programming efforts in our culture are working aggressively, passively, and consistently. Since the majority of these influences are based on profitability not only has our society become influenced to think attractive is better but it has also shown favor to the attractive population.

The Reality of the Relationship Scale

Reality can be candid. When it comes to physical appearance the majority of people tend to start out with others that are so-called in their scale bracket as determined by our younger generation. It is a very sensitive subject to discuss however; the realism of it speaks for itself. For example, if you took a look at several couples of people that were in newly developed relationships and evaluated their looks you will find what many people in society have a hard time admitting to. In fact, this is one of the first few publications that cover this topic. Here is how the world is operating.

What will most people think when they see a large overweight man that appears to not take care of himself in a relationship together with a very attractive woman that is in shape? Most people will wonder how the man was able to achieve in getting this woman and many will automatically assume he has a lot of wealth. This goes the same if the situation is vice versa for an attractive man compared to a very overweight woman. Most people tend to always think there is some logical reason they are in a committed relationship. When in fact it could be because of the pure essence of genuine, kind love.

The Positive Opportunity to Losing Weight

Now that you understand the realism of many people's subconscious minds from an early age it is important for you to understand your opportunity. If a man or woman has the opportunity to expand their capabilities of possibilities of attractive potential partners why do we not have more people in today's world in shape?

The reason is two-fold:

1) They are taught that this thinking is bad, which can sometimes lead to a lack of motivation to be fit. Since we are taught that beauty on the inside is only what is important it discredits the justifications of reasoning to strive for fitness in today's world.

and

2) Many people may not realize or understand how the effectiveness of physical attraction will play a role in their life when it comes to the attractiveness of others, therefore, parents normally do not use this principle for motivation to be fit. When in fact it plays a huge factor in how others are attracted to us physically and should be one of the many reasons why people need to be even more motivated. Since many of our minds work very visual it may be beneficial for us to see how the numbers factor would work if using the scale factor that is practiced by much of our younger society.

3 Reasons WHY to Take On The World and Master Fitness

1) Why We Strive
2) Projecting Visual Images Become Real
3) It's YOUR Opportunity - The Reason You Should

1) Why We Strive

Understand what is taking place when you are getting in shape. One of the deepest human desires is to be loved and respected. It is a natural need we have as people and without it, there would be much emptiness. It confines from our children, our achievements, and our desires to succeed in life. We strive for excellence and the ability to satisfy our loved ones and create a satisfying life for them. The desire to care for our young would still be there as a bearing of emptiness if we did not have children in our lives. Our desire to feel a level of importance deep down is a priority that is at a different surface level with many at different times in people's lives. Regardless of what timeline in life you are at, you deserve to be all you can and achieve the happiness you so deserve.

2) Projections

When you transform your body to be in top shape you are going through one of the most complex psychological experiences the mind can go through. There is a series of changes that take place that will affect the many attributes of one's character in a positive way. Not only are these changes taking place in our minds but our bodies are sending the messages of how we feel to others. When someone is in shape their body is projecting signals when they appear in different environments.

These signals are what adds to a person with an attractive body to be much more attractive than a person without an attractive body. Fitness in retrospect projects several visuals that send signals with no words required. As we receive these visuals we translate them in our head as several things.

We assume a nice lean body must signify the following as, discipline, productiveness, and that the person respects himself or herself which in turn is confidence. This confidence is then perceived into initial attraction and regardless of what level of attractiveness someone is at, they can naturally improve their overall attractiveness just by being fit.

The images of projection work in almost every aspect we can think of in how our appearance is to others. It signifies a combination of attractiveness combined with confidence. Much of this is without awareness of reality. For example, one of the key attributes that females want in a male is height. Statistics have proven that women generally prefer an attractive mate that is somewhat tall. This is an example of how the images of projection works since studies show the reason is that height tends to signify good genes subliminally. In addition, it is natural for the height of a male to be viewed as a good primate, which in turn is why women are attracted to tall men subconsciously without realizing why. With all of our bodies appearances and attributes weight is one thing that we have control over. **For men that are not tall:** If you cannot control the height that your body is capable of growing, take charge of what you can control. If women's subconscious minds are working in the background relating height to good genes then it is your responsibility to reflect the highest image of projection as possible by taking care of your body and maintaining the best shape you possibly can. Now that you understand this it is your time for a change by projecting your visual images of who you really are to become a reality.

3) It's YOUR Opportunity - "The Reason Why You Should"

This is the reason why everyone should desire and start making the changes you need to reach the fitness level you desire. You have the opportunity to raise your level of attractiveness and project your image to others around you without words. There are limited physical things that you have the power to change to modify your appearance such as the clothes you wear, etc. Weight is one of the most influential factors that has one of the highest impacts when it comes to images of projection. Although it is one of the more difficult attributes you can change it can also be one of your best attributes as you build the body of your dreams. When you achieve this you will have one of the most effective feelings of accomplishments that the human mind can achieve, to feel good about yourself and be perceived to others that you are in control of your life.

This helps to satisfy that natural human desire and is conducive to assisting the mind to be in a confident state, which can lead to improving the many things and paths you choose in life.
Simply Put
"Fitness will give you the opportunity on how you decide to take on the world which is exactly the reason why you

should."

ACTION STEPS:

1) Admit the truth to yourself of how society views being overweight. Realize that being fit signifies discipline.

2) Decide if you want to embrace and change to live a more fulfilling life by simply asking yourself what would make you happier?

3) The images of projection work in your favor. Accept the fact that physical appearance is the initial determining factor that sparks physical attraction before getting acquainted with others. Decide if you want to give yourself the upper hand by magnifying your appearance to attract a whole new category of attractive people for potential relationships and every opportunity that life throws at you.

CONCLUSION

It is human nature to act out distinctly in different scenarios. For example, people with absolutely no money may not be as confident going into an environment with others that have success and wealth. It is normal for someone that may not have the experience to feel intimidation and a sense of not belonging. I personally have witnessed this process from being on both sides of the fence to go from having nothing to having everything I desire. It gives you a new confidence level that is simply indescribable and makes you feel capable to socialize with anybody.

Losing weight is no different and is in every way

comparable to life. In order to fit in today's world to the extent of your fullest potential of confidence, you can achieve this feeling. You get one chance at life. Unless you have a personal reincarnation ticket you have one shot to live this life to its fullest potential. Have a talk with yourself. Tell this to yourself and make <u>you</u> realize this. It is this powerful motivational thinking that will turn into action.

"The one individual that determines if we are successful at anything is you."

THIS SHIRT IS 4 YEARS OLD - smh

I was 29 and I remember coming out of the restroom at a new popular sports bar that served food and drinks.

I was just starting to lose weight. I was a handsome fellow but like most people weight didn't do me any justice.

I was down to around 255lbs, wearing a suit jacket with a cream low cut turtleneck. I had bought the cream color shirt 4 years prior at Men's Wearhouse because I saw it and fell in love with it but they didn't have my size. I figured I would lose enough weight to fit into it one day and took a gamble.

It had been hanging in my closet and I was happy I finally got to wear it.

As I came out of the restroom there were two women standing close by the walk area that led to the bar. I thought they were waiting in line for the bar area but it turns out they were just standing and talking.

It's almost as if they were waiting to talk to me when I came out of the restroom.

We made eye contact and it would have been awkward if we didn't say anything because their focus was directly in front of me.

One of them said, "Hey, that shirt is working for you. You are well put together, that color looks good on you."

All I could say was, "thanks, this shirt is 4 years old."

Rather than elaborating about my weight loss story, I kind of awkwardly froze after that. You see I wasn't used to getting compliments about my appearance as well as being flirted with directly.

I couldn't believe it was happening and till this day I laugh because all I could say was, "thanks it's 4 years old!"

What was I thinking?! I wasn't, because I was not used to being approached like that and was caught off guard.

I remember the awkwardness smiles from all three of us for those few seconds. I didn't stick around long and said "thank you" and politely walk away.

I was not interested in those women but it was a good feeling to receive a compliment.
I realized that all my hard work is starting to pay off and be noticed.

You see, when you decide to pursue your weight loss journey people are going to begin to treat you differently.

You are going to start receiving compliments and if you are not used to receiving such compliments you may not know how to react to them.

It's almost like you want to do a double-take at times and look behind you to see if people are smiling at you or the person behind you.

But it will be in fact "you" they will be smiling at.

Like it or not, it is a judgemental society and people will treat you differently as you begin shedding pounds.

I used to think of it as superficial and was not sure how to handle it.

But think of it as your reward. All your hard work that you put in. Whether if you are married or in a relationship, you can still enjoy being treated well with pride.

People will treat you differently and this will boost your self-esteem.

It will reinforce your confidence.

It will be motivating for you to work even harder.

The cold hard truth is, whether if it's an attraction or simply people just giving you respect because they see a person that takes care of themselves... people will start to treat you differently.

When it happens to you, just remember to say something better than, "this shirt is 4 years old."

Chapter 14

Evolving Routine to an Effortless Health Lifestyle

The Exercise Momentum Cycle

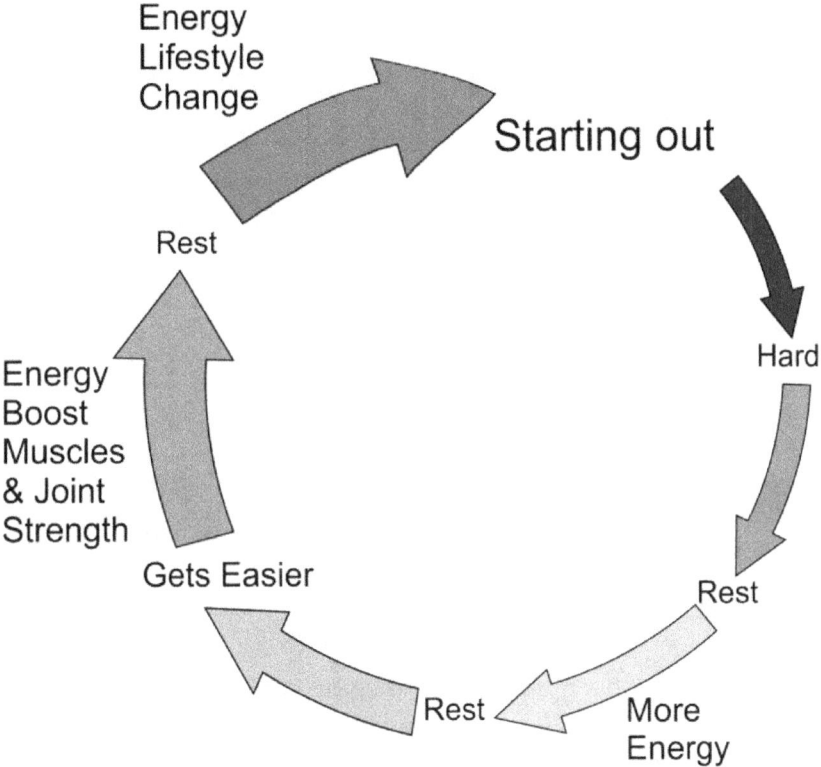

Congratulations

So this is it. This is the stage you reach that you pretty much achieved the level of fitness you desire or you pretty much are on the path to where you got this in the bag. If you have not achieved this level yet here is what you can expect.

Remember when you were first studying for your driver's license exam? Yes as a young teenager you might recall all the thought process you needed to operate and become a licensed driver. It required study and effort. It required your full focus to learn the motions of the vehicle, the brakes, the controls, and acceleration. Pretty soon you progressed and got to the point when you get in the car and drive you no longer have to think about it. Sometimes you can get in the vehicle and end up at your location and not even remember driving there. Driving becomes almost like walking, just an everyday motion you do without much thought. This is exactly how it is once you reach the level of evolving routine to an effortless health lifestyle.

If you have already reached this point of success then congratulations! Evolving into diet and exercise routines to the point where you do it without thinking about it is the key to a lifetime achievement of fitness.

Most people have a false perception of living a healthy lifestyle that it is hard. When in reality it is only embracing the change at the beginning that is difficult. Once you pass this initial phase and develop health habits it becomes easy. Just as learning all the traffic laws, signs, and focusing on a vehicle's movements this is similar to the fitness lifestyle. Once you learn all the do's and don'ts of eating and become accustomed to exercising as part of your daily routine then your life will change forever.

Learning all the fundamentals for anything, in the beginning, is always going to take effort but once you become a pro at your health you will love the feeling when you get there. It becomes easier to go to the gym when needed and make the right food choices. It is no longer a shock to your body and you can accomplish more without as much struggle. The benefit of this level is being able to take your body to a new level of the fitness goals you desire. This is the window of opportunity for you to focus. This is the time to concentrate on many of the perfections you strive for. Muscle tone, definition, abs, and symmetry are all in your reach. It is a time for the evolution of how you chose to live your life.

The Delusional Plateau

In the very beginning stage of weight loss, you will find that much of the initial weight will fall off fairly quickly if you are putting in a lot of effort. This is the case especially if you are obese and have a lot of excessive weight. The closer you get to your ideal body weight the slower weight will start to come off. When you get to your final pounds that you need to lose this is where you start to reach a plateau.

Do not worry if you are not losing as much weight as fast as you were in the beginning. You're still making progress and your body is going through its natural survival mechanisms to try and keep the last bit of the weight on. Nature has its rules to protect you. For these rules to be broken, it is going to take extra effort when we get to the bottom layer of fat. Here is how it works and why we hit plateaus towards the end.

Let's say for example you weighed 300 lbs and are 150 lbs overweight. If you lost 140 lbs then that would be a result equivalent to 40% of your entire body weight. That is nearly half of you! Losing the last 10% when your body's survival mechanisms have kicked in is generally going to be much more difficult than losing almost half your body weight. Don't worry, it will come and you can do it. It's simply going to take a little longer to get the last few pounds of weight off and I consider that one of those good problems in life to have.

As you evolve to this advanced level of fitness these are the times you will have to shock your body, nervous system, and muscles to new levels. While it may seem like you are on a plateau just remember this is the delusional plateau phase and you will still achieve your goals. Just keep going.

You Are On Top Of The World

When you arrive at this point you will feel that you are on top of the world. It took such a long path to get here. Everything that was working against you, you conquered. However, now is the time you must maintain. It is much harder to climb a mountain in the beginning however staying on top of a mountain does not require as much effort as you are no longer scaling up.

You no longer have to go into calorie deficit every single day. Only a couple of days a week or two days at a time if you need fine-tuning. You will find that maintenance and upkeep is much easier than having to rebuild your entire body. You begin to eat more for the reason of how it makes you feel afterward versus eating for how it makes you feel while eating it. It is similar to drinking coffee in the mornings. Generally, we drink coffee because of how it makes us feel, not because of the taste. When you start becoming attentive to how your body is feeling after consuming certain foods you start to develop a better awareness to want to be more health-conscious without thinking about it. Soon you start to notice the sugar crashes and low energy that result from junk foods as well as how nutritional foods make you feel energetic. Your new sense of awareness of how food makes you feel will start to become effortless the same as your workouts. Your body is how you live this lifetime. Make it count.

Some days you will find that not only your workouts progress but so does your natural muscle tone. You start to find new strengths and abilities you never thought you had before. It almost becomes like an addictive process that cannot be stopped. The compliments keep coming and the way life treats you differently is such a game-changer that it makes you never want to go back to your old ways. You start to crave the "better mood" feeling resulting from good nutrition and if you happen to miss several days of the gym from being on a vacation or not able to work out you can't wait to get right back into your fitness ritual. This is the point where you have reached your destination. This is when you feel on top of the world.

Stay there.

Feel this great feeling everyday life allows you to and never go back. It is just too wonderful and you deserve to feel this way for life.

Now that you have reached the near end of this book let's recap over everything you have learned. This is the best way to ensure you absorbed much of its content so you can begin losing weight immediately and achieve the body you've always wanted.

Chapter 1 First - Which Motivation Level Are You? - You have begun to understand the different levels of motivation. You know much of the reasoning from a logical standpoint on the foundation of what motivates people to lose weight and the basic reasons for their motivations. You learned to understand your own motivation and ask yourself what is it that motivates you as well as how you can level up.

Chapter 2 The Hunger Pain Drug - You learned mind techniques you can use to curb your hunger cravings. This is where you learned to realize how food cravings are like a drug and in order to battle the cravings you have to battle them before it's too late. The key to battling cravings of poor food choices is finding a balance and avoiding the hunger pains. Remember to not let yourself become too hungry so that it will result in you making better decisions about what you eat. Remember the importance of controlling your environment of influences so that mirror neurons to mimic will affect you in a positive way.

Chapter 3 Two Steps Forward, Never Two Steps Back - This is where you learned about the weekly step system as a way to measure your weekly progress. You learned the concept of making progress is similar as if you were swimming a long distance and keep poking your head out of the water to see how far you have swam. We learned the importance of having clarity of our goals keeps our mindset focused. This is where you covered the importance to write everything that you eat in a food journal. This gives us health awareness of what we are putting inside our bodies which will result in better eating choices.

Chapter 4 Weight Loss Desires - What You Want - We learned about our constant desires of what drives us and how powerful it is to utilize your thoughts to your advantage to inspire you. You learned how to utilize the way your mind works so that you can think about vacations, and other upcoming events so that you can always be striving for that high school skinny mentality.

Chapter 5 Shrinking Your Stomach Process - This is where you learned about the shrinking of your stomach process and how in actuality your stomach does not technically shrink however since it stretches less you can develop the feeling to feel satisfied as a gradual process. The end result will involve you to lose many pounds and physically your stomach will shrink while your internal stomach will become used to not being stretched on a consistent basis. Developing the ability to get passed this temporary discomfort phase as a new habit is key to your weight loss success. Remember the discomfort is temporary and it will take less effort as time passes. Remember to drink water and fill yourself with healthy food choices when needed.

Chapter 6 In the Zone - You learned about being at the crossroads for many of the daily decisions you will be faced with every day. This is where you heard about the howling dog story of how the nail did not hurt him bad enough. You learned about how bad programming starts early in life and how to stay motivated by going into the zone of fitness which involves overcoming all of societies subliminal messages that are constantly trying to make us unhealthy. Not being in the zone is generally a result of life and society's bad programming but in order to win the battle, we have to overcome the world's modern-day conditioning.

Chapter 7 Super Weight Loss Focus - You learned mind techniques and the power of simplifying your life so you can be focused. Similar to the pairing of socks when doing laundry the sooner you get started, the easier it becomes as you begin to eliminate and simply start making progress. Everything always seems hard in the beginning when in reality it will become simple.

We discussed the same way how it takes time to be submerged in uncomfortable pool water is similar when getting over the uncomfortable period when losing weight. You learned how the progression of time makes the focus required to lose weight easier and it's simply about getting started to get over the uncomfortable period. Losing weight is simply the choice of deciding whether you are going to go into a calorie deficit and how many days per week you are going to do it.

We also discussed how to not waste your daily deposit of time and that the investment you make for a healthy lifestyle gives you very high returns. This return on your investment is many more years of life which is why the time for change is now. You are worth it.

Chapter 8 The Right Partner - This is where we learned

about how the person we choose to spend the most time with will influence our healthy lifestyle whether it's good or bad. We have to make the decision how strong we are going to be whether if it's to deal with resistance or get our partner to join us.

We realized that ultimately that it is better if our partner joins us in the fitness lifestyle and if they don't we must be prepared for how we are going to handle it however we must recognize the decision of our life's health belongs to nobody but ourselves.

Chapter 9 The Social Event We learned the four aspects that make the difference when we attend life's social events.

- Alcohol
- Socialization
- Influence
- Celebration

We also learned that we must have these social events to keep life interesting and if we must have them, then we have to make them worth celebrating. And that it is better to have more celebrations healthy to be able to have more celebrations in life.

Chapter 10 Activation Your Energy Source for Life - This where you learned about the different times you work out as well as the different analogies you can use to get started to boost your energy level and get warmed up. We also discussed how you play golf with better golfers and how important it is to surround yourself with positive people for your performance.

Use Psychological Visuals:
This is where you learned how to instantly feel better and how to start prescribing yourself an energy boost. How to take advantage of all the mental visuals to warm up to get the blood pumping and get your body moving.
Remember how to keep your mind motivated to kill cardio time as well as the different techniques to keep your mind focused to get you through your cardio sessions by using psychological visuals.

Chapter 11 Weight Loss After Pregnancy - This is where we covered the examples of the different levels of fitness moms and their mindsets to better understand their different motivation levels. We went through the reasons why it is wise to lead by example and how important it is for moms to be their healthiest. How the parent filter works and how habits of lifestyle are passed down. Remember to not lose sight of being a healthy mom but also a healthy grandma!

Chapter 12 Using Supplements to Boost Your Mental Motivation - In this chapter we discussed how you can use supplements to boost your motivation as a temporary boost. We also covered the importance of proper massage to assist with maintenance, especially for resistance training. Remember that illegal supplements do not make any sense, especially if your living does not depend on your athletic ability and that longevity will thank you with many healthy years to come.

Chapter 13 The Cold Hard Truth - This is where we covered how we live in a judgmental society however, it is important to remember, "You are a vibration of your own frequency that you decide to project to the world." We have to embrace the fact that fitness has an impact on jobs, relationships and many different aspects of life. We also covered how there is good and bad judgment. This means it is our choice of which judgmental side of the fence that you will end up on. We discussed the benefits of being on the different parts of the spectrum of judgment since people can also judge for you looking fit and attractive. Your glowing personality combined with strong fitness health is what is sexy and you deserve to feel this way.

Chapter 14 Evolving Routine to an Effortless Lifestyle - The exercise momentum cycle will boost your energy for life because it's similar to a merry go round in a city park. Once you start pushing and turning it momentum kicks in and it gets easier. You will get moving towards your weight loss goals and shed off many pounds. Then after experiencing a great feeling of accomplishment generally there will be a time you will get to the delusional plateau. Remember this is one of those good problems to have. The reason it is a delusional stage because progress seems to slow down as far as pounds lost however, remember you are still making progress.

Don't forget to shock your body with new challenges. This is when you don't stop and this is where you need to remember to "floor it" an expression to press the gas all the way down to the floorboard. Put that pedal to the medal to drive right across the finish line to your weight loss goals and floor it.

Now that you have arrived at this feeling of being on top of the world remember to eat to feel better and think about how you will feel after you consume certain foods. Develop the awareness that with the right mindset fitness is an evolving routine to an effortless lifestyle.

Giving Back

At this point, you have realized the actions you have taken
have helped you to take control of your life. The fact that
you have changed the way you think and how your mind
works you have figured out the source of your decisions
and how to use this knowledge to control your body's
physique. Now that you are controlling the source of your
decisions with your mental strength, help teach others. Tell
them about this book. Explain the principles that will help
them. It takes a certain person to have the ability to take
control of their destiny and if you have achieved what you
worked so hard for then you have what it takes to continue
to be prosperous at everything you do. Do not let your gift
of knowledge go unused and give back. You have the
ability to make a difference in people's lives. Influence and
encourage others. Set the standards of hope and lead by
example. Take control of paving the path to help clear the
skies and help lead others to their fitness destination.

When you become super fit, healthy and attractive what is
the point of it all? Who cares if you do not have a good
soul? How you make others feel around you is what is
important. There is a certain energy and vibe you will
project as a very fit person. If you make others feel
envious, insecure or not very good about themselves then
you have done all this for nothing. Life is about passing the
torch of success and giving back so we can continue to
develop and grow together.

And when you stand in front of somebody and project the
love and peaceful energy off to help and uplift and inspire

others then this is true success and you have reached the ultimate fitness goal.

Congratulations

Love is Strength

-Gilbert Quinones

THE UNDERDOG FRESHMAN - Never Give Up

IN 1992 I WAS AN OVERWEIGHT 14 YR OLD FRESHMAN AND IT WAS LAST PERIOD IN SOCCER.

When school started, the first two weeks were HELL because coach Streckel told us, "If you don't like to run, don't be in soccer."

Coach was around his mid 40's.. he literally had Popeye calves and could outrun anybody on the team and would many times lead in sprints.

For practice, we always had to run laps and as the chubby kid, everyone thought I would quit after the first day. I wanted to but didn't because I knew I was an underdog.

There was a mixture of all grade levels in soccer period, including freshmen with juniors and seniors. I felt so honored to have a class with older kids.

After two weeks, I began to gain respect from the other students and even some of the seniors. Being accepted and respected made me feel noble.

During practice, while everyone was running past me, I would just keep jogging to keep my body moving while trying to control my breathing.

Sometimes, the older fit kids would run beside me and say, "Gilbert.. breath in through your nose and out through your mouth." 🐶

Two weeks went by and I thought I was getting the hang of being overweight and running laps for soccer until one Monday, something happened.

I walked into the locker room and felt this day was different. Coach had a SERIOUS look on his face and I immediately knew something was wrong.

He said, "Get dressed fast and get to the field."

It turned out something bad happened the previous weekend at soccer practice (I wasn't there). That previous weekend after practice was over it got dark and a few unnamed players stuck around and turned on the stadium lights at the old Ave E field costing the school a $400.00 electric bill for ONE NIGHT.

They were not supposed to stay after practice, turn on the stadium lights or play into the night leaving the lights on. When the school told coach what happened he got the heat for it and he was pissed.

I wasn't there but that did not matter. That Monday EVERYONE in soccer class was in trouble.

We got to the field and my adrenaline was pumping because I knew we were about to be punished.

Coach said...

"You boys are going to run the entire hour and you are going to run hard."

"You better not stop unless you are puking. If I see one person stop, unless you stopped to puke, we are going to do this every day until you get it right."

We started running and immediately my heart was already beating fast because I was scared.

I was afraid I was going to let the team down. Coach could see all of us running around the field and I did not know how I was going to make it without stopping. I DID NOT want to be the one to let the team down.

After 20 minutes I remember the bright sun and it being so freaking hot! My leg muscles were aching so bad. My side was hurting and I was trying to control my (in through nose, out through mouth) breathing but it wasn't working out

Some of the seniors saw I was struggling to stay running and they would occasionally run beside me.

I tried so hard to not let tears run down my face. No one really noticed because we were sweating so much.

As much as it hurt and as much as I wanted to stop, I didn't. I just kept thinking.. if I stop, everybody is going to have to do this again tomorrow.

30 minutes went by and it felt like forever.

40 minutes went by and it became unbearable.

50 minutes went by and it was excruciating.

I couldn't wait till 1-hour hit and I felt like I was going to collapse on the ground and die.

FINALLY, 1 hour came and I never thought I would be so happy to hear that whistle blow.

Hands on my knees and then down to the ground I went. I was breathing so out of control but I was so glad it was over.

I was exhausted but made it. When we got back to the locker room I saw coach standing by the doorway. As I was about to walk inside he stopped me, looked right at me and said,

"Gilbert, I know you weren't there. Not everyone was. But that's the way life is sometimes. Good job today."

It was the greatest feeling to hear him say that. That punishment scarred me in probably the healthiest way possible.

Curveballs in life come in all forms. Many will cause you much pain. Sometimes it's not your fault and you still have to deal with it.

Thank you to everyone who always kept encouraging me and to coach Streckel for teaching a very hard but valuable lesson.

I wish you all the best of luck in dealing with any obstacles that may get in your way.

May you gain strength and honor to deal with any pain that tries to get you to quit.

As long as there is still air in your lungs.

Never. Give. Up.

-Gilbert

The following have been an influence in my life and have made a difference to make this book be possible in some way. Whether pertaining to fitness, gave me words of encouragement or a positive influence in my life that motivated me to be better.

Special Thanks to:
Teresa & Darrell Cowan, Julius Quinones, Robert Quinones, Cathy & Bill Purdy, Joseph Cowan, Camryn Little, Jon Ray, Susan Quinones, Tom & Hermalinda Sandifer, Steve & Patricia Meadows, Jason Witmer, George Farley, Dr Robert Caridi, Avedis Garcia, Patrick Maxam, Michael McGehee, Jeffrey Lopez, Carlos Lopez, Elaine Quinones, Luis Guzman, Mike Hrostoski, Dane Maxwell, David Cantu, Curtis Smith, Roc Garza, Paul Doyle, Catherine Stewart, Ebun Muhammad, Jonathan Delgado, Dr William Perry, Chuck Strasburg, Julius Zatopek, Wally Wilson, Buzzy Knapp, Richard Filip, Robert Herrings, John Terry, Bill Phillips, Dave Cordoncillo, Cheryl Fairbanks, Mike & Denise Zehr, Odessa Fernandez, Maxwell Ochieng, Derek Anderson, Coach Streckel, Michael Wheat, Felix Chien, Harry Haung.